A Text Atlas of Nail Disorders

A Text Atlas of Nail Disorders

Diagnosis and Treatment

Robert Baran, MD
Nail Disease Centre
Cannes, France

Rodney Dawber, MA, MB, ChB, FRCP
Consultant Dermatologist
Churchill Hospital, Oxford, UK

Eckart Haneke, MD
Director, Ferdinand Sauerbruch Hospital
Wuppertal, Germany

Antonella Tosti, MD
Associate Professor of Dermatology, University of Bologna
Bologna, Italy

With contributions from:
Ivan Bristow
Podiatrist, Churchill Hospital
Oxford, UK

MARTIN DUNITZ

© Martin Dunitz 1996

First published in the United Kingdom in 1996 by
Martin Dunitz Ltd
The Livery House
7-9 Pratt Street
London NW1 0AE

Reprinted 1997

A CIP record for this book is available from the British Library.

ISBN 1-85317-201-4

Composition by Scribe Design, Gillingham, Kent
Originated, printed and bound in Singapore by Kyodo Printing Co (S'pore) Pte Ltd

Contents

Preface   vii

1   **Science of the nail apparatus and relationship to foot function**   1

Structure   1
Microscopic anatomy   3
Blood and nerve supply   4
Nail dynamics   5
The nails in childhood and old age   6
Foot function   7
Foot shape   10
Footwear   10

2   **Nail configuration abnormalities**   17

Clubbing (Hippocratic fingers)   17
Koilonychia (spoon-shaped nails)   23
Transverse overcurvature   26
Dolichonychia (long nails)   30
Brachyonychia (short nails)   33
Parrot beak nails   35
Hook and claw-like nails   35

Micro- and macronychia and polydactyly   37
Worn down and shiny nails   39
Anonychia and onychatrophy   42

3   **Modifications of nail surface**   49

Longitudinal lines   49
Herringbone nails   53
Transverse lines   53
Pitting and rippling   58
Trachyonychia (rough nails)   60
Onychoschizia (lamellar splitting)   63

4   **Nail plate and soft tissue abnormalities**   67

Onycholysis   67
Onychomadesis and shedding   71
Hypertrophy and subungual hyperkeratosis   72
Splinter haemorrhages and subungual haematoma   80
Dorsal and ventral pterygium   84

5   Periungual tissue disorders   89
Paronychia   89
Ragged cuticles and 'hang nail'   93
Painful dorsolateral fissures of the
finger tip   96
Tumours and swellings   98
Pustules   121

6   Nail consistency   133
Fragile, brittle and soft nails   133

**7   Nail colour changes
(chromonychia)**   139
Leukonychia (white nail)   140
Melanonychia (brown/black nail)   147
Other discolorations   153

**8   Onychomycosis and its
treatment**   155
Onychomycosis due to
dermatophytes   155
Onychomycosis due to
non-dermatophytic moulds   165
Candida onychomycosis   167

**9   Traumatic disorders of the nail
with special reference to the
toes and painful nail**   169
Major trauma   169
Repeated microtrauma of the nail
apparatus   172
The painful nail   193

**10   Treatment of common nail
disorders**   199
Brittle nails   199
Cosmetic treatment of nail
dystrophies   200
Acute paronychia   201
Blistering distal dactylitis   202
Chronic paronychia   202
Onycholysis   202
Psoriasis   203
Lichen planus   204
Twenty nail dystrophy   204
Yellow nail syndrome   204
Onychogryphosis   204
Nail biting and
onychotillomania   205
Periungual warts   205

Index   207

Preface

Patients do not present with diseases but with specific symptoms or signs i.e. dis-ease! Most textbooks in clinical medicine are written and organized in relation to disease classification. Because nail apparatus problems produce distinct, often very vividly obvious signs, we thought that since many clinicians find nail abnormalities difficult to diagnose, it might be of use to produce a text atlas emphasizing differential diagnosis. It is particularly aimed at those who see nail problems in their practice and may not be fully conversant with the subtleties of nail apparatus diagnosis. This type of book evidently requires colour illustrations and we very much hope that those selected are sufficiently clear and diverse to aid diagnosis.

This is not a reference book; we have simply provided lists of further useful reading. If the reader requires more detailed information we recommend: *Diseases of the Nails and Their Management*, 2nd edn (Blackwell Scientific Publishers: Oxford 1994) — all the editors of this text atlas contributed to this reference book.

Robert Baran
Rodney Dawber
Eckart Haneke
Antonella Tosti

1 Science of the nail apparatus and relationship to foot function

The anatomy and physiology of the nail apparatus on the hand may be considered in isolation; however the nail apparatus on the toes must always be considered in relation to toe and foot structure and function. Many disorders of nails are directly due to functional faults in the foot; alternatively, diseases of the nail apparatus may be modified by alterations in digital or foot shape or movement.

> **The nail is a very important 'tool' and adds great subtlety and protection to the digit**

The nail apparatus develops from the primitive epidermis. The main function of the nail apparatus is to produce a strong, relatively inflexible nail plate over the dorsal surface of the end of each digit. The nail plate acts as a protective covering for the fingertip; by exerting counter pressure over the volar skin and pulp, the relatively flat nail plate adds to the precision and delicacy of both the ability to pick up small objects and many other subtle finger functions, e.g. counter pressure against the plantar skin and pulp prevents the heaping up of the distal soft tissue. Finger nails typically cover approximately one-fifth of the dorsal surface, whilst on the great toe, the nail may cover up to 50% of the dorsum of the digit. Toe nails and finger nails have varying shapes and curvature. This is partly controlled by the shape of the underlying distal phalangeal bones.

Structure

The component parts of the nail apparatus are shown diagrammatically in Figure 1.1a, b and in biopsy in 1.1c. The rectangular nail plate is the largest structure, resting on and firmly attached to the nail bed and the underlying bones, less firm proximally, apart from the posterolateral corners. Approximately one-quarter of the nail is covered by the proximal nail fold whilst a narrow margin of the sides of the nail plate is often occluded by the lateral nail folds. Underlying the proximal part of the nail is the white lunula (syn. half-moon lunule); this area represents the most distal region of the matrix. The natural shape of the free margin of the nail is the same as the contour of the distal border on the lunula. The nail plate

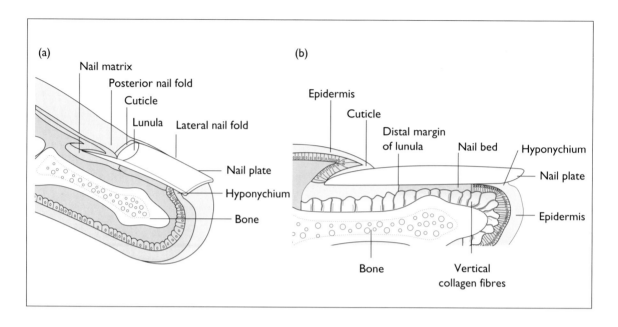

(a)

Nail matrix
Posterior nail fold
Cuticle
Lunula   Lateral nail fold
Nail plate
Hyponychium
Bone

(b)

Epidermis
Cuticle
Distal margin of lunula   Nail bed   Hyponychium
Nail plate
Epidermis
Bone   Vertical collagen fibres

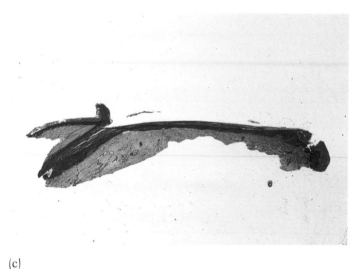

(c)

Figure 1.1

(**a**) and (**b**) Nail apparatus structures; (**c**) longitudinal nail biopsy orientated to equate with (**b**).

distal to the lunula is usually pink due to its translucency which allows the redness of the vascular nail bed to be seen through it. The proximal nail fold has two epithelial surfaces, dorsal and ventral; at the junction of the two the cuticle projects distally onto the nail surface. The lateral nail folds are in continuity with the skin on the sides of the digit laterally, and medially they are joined by the nail bed.

The nail matrix can be subdivided into proximal and distal sections, the latter underlying the nail plate to the distal border of the lunula; some texts prefer the terms dorsal and intermediate matrix respectively. It is now generally considered that the nail bed contributes to the deep surface of the nail plate (ventral matrix), though this deep component plays little part in the functional integrity of the nail plate in its distal part. At the point of separation of the nail plate from the nail bed, the proximal part of the hyponychium may be modified as the solehorn. Beyond the solehorn region the hyponychium terminates at the distal nail groove; the tip of the digit beyond this ridge assumes the structure of the epidermis elsewhere.

When the attached nail plate is viewed from above several distinct areas may be visible, such as the proximal lunula and the larger pink zone. On close examination two further distal zones can often be identified, the distal yellowish-white margin and immediately proximal to this the onychodermal band. This latter band is a barely perceptible narrow transverse band 0.5–1.5 mm wide. The exact anatomical basis for the onychodermal (onychocorneal) band is not known but it appears to have a separate blood supply from that of the main body of the nail bed; if the tip of the finger is pressed firmly, the band and an area just proximal to it blanch, and if the pressure is repeated several times the band reddens.

Microscopic anatomy

Nail fold

The proximal nail fold is similar in structure to the adjacent skin but is normally devoid of dermatoglyphic markings and sebaceous glands. From the distal area of the proximal nail fold the cuticle reflects onto the surface of the nail plate; it is composed of modified

stratum corneum and serves to protect the structures at the base of the nail, particularly the germinative matrix, from environmental insults such as irritants, allergens and bacterial and fungal pathogens.

Nail matrix

The proximal and distal nail matrix (syn. dorsal and intermediate respectively) is the area which produces the major part of the nail plate. As in the epidermis of the skin, the matrix possesses a dividing basal layer producing keratinocytes which differentiate, harden, die and contribute to the nail plate, which is thus analogous to the epidermal stratum corneum. The nail matrix keratinocytes mature and keratinize without keratohyalin (granular layer) formation. Apart from this, the detailed cytological changes seen in the matrix epithelium under the electron microscope are essentially the same as in the epidermis.

The nail matrix contains melanocytes in the lowest two cell layers and these donate pigment to keratinocytes. Under normal circumstances pigment is not visible in the nail plate of white Caucasoid individuals, but many Negroid subjects show patchy melanogenesis as linear longitudinal pigmented bands.

> **On the great toes, the nail matrix sits like a saddle on the distal phalanx**

Nail bed

This consists of an epidermal part (ventral matrix) and the underlying dermis closely apposed to the periosteum of the distal phalanx. There is no subcutaneous fat layer in the nail bed, although scattered dermal fat cells may be visible microscopically. The nail bed epidermal layer (sterile ventral matrix) is usually no more than two or three cells thick, and the transitional zone from living keratinocyte to dead ventral nail plate cell is abrupt, occurring in the space of one horizontal cell layer. As the cells differentiate they are incorporated into the ventral surface of the nail plate and move distally with this layer.

The nail bed dermal collagen is mainly orientated vertically, being directly attached to phalangeal periosteum and the epidermal basal lamina. Within the connective tissue network lie blood vessels, lymphatics, a fine network of elastic fibres and scattered fat cells; at the distal margin, eccrine sweat glands have been seen.

Nail plate

The nail plate is made of three horizontal layers: a thin dorsal lamina, the thicker intermediate lamina and a ventral layer from the nail bed. Microscopically, it is composed of flattened squamous cells closely apposed to each other. In older age groups, acidophilic masses are occasionally seen: the so-called pertinax bodies.

The nail plate is rich in calcium, found as the phosphate in hydroxyapatite crystals; it is bound to phospholipids intracellularly. The relevance of other metals which are present in smaller amounts, such as copper, manganese, zinc and iron, is not exactly known. Calcium exists in a concentration of 0.1% by weight, 10 times greater than in hair. Calcium does not significantly contribute to the hardness of the nail. Nail hardness is mainly due to the high sulphur matrix protein, which contrasts with the relatively soft keratin of the epidermis. The normal curvature of the nail relates to the shape of the underlying phalangeal bone to which the nail plate is directly bonded via the vertical

connective tissue attached between the subungual epithelium and the periosteum.

Blood and nerve supply

> **The nail apparatus has a magnificent blood supply with many anastomoses**

There is a rich arterial blood supply to the nail bed and matrix derived from paired digital arteries (Figure 1.2a, b and c). The main supply passes into the pulp space of the distal phalanx before reaching the dorsum of the digit. The volar digital nerves (Figure 1.2c) are similarly important in providing nerves to the deep nail apparatus structures. An accessory blood supply arises further back on the digit and does not enter the pulp space. There are two main arterial arches (proximal and distal) supplying the nail bed and matrix, formed from anastomoses of the branches of the digital arteries. In the event of damage to the main supply in the pulp space, such as may occur with infection or scleroderma, there may be sufficient blood from the accessory vessels to permit normal growth of the nail.

There is a capillary loop system to the whole of the nail fold, but the loops to the roof and matrix are flatter than those below the exposed nail. There are many arteriovenous anastomoses below the nail – glomus bodies, which are concerned with heat regulation. Glomus bodies are important in maintaining acral circulation under cold conditions – arterioles constrict with cold but glomus bodies dilate. The nail beds of fingers and toes contain such bodies (93–501 per cm^2). Each glomus is an encapsulated oval organ 300 μm long, made up of a tortuous vessel uniting an artery and venule, a nerve supply and a capsule; also within the capsule are many cholinergic muscle cells.

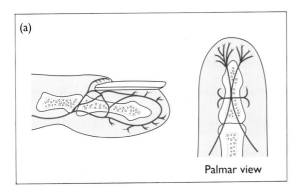

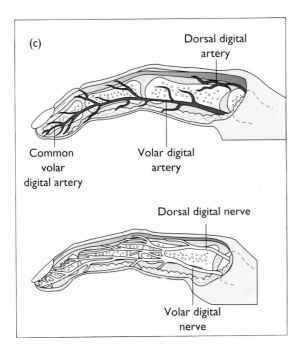

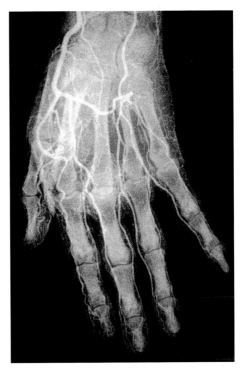

(b)

Figure 1.2

Digital blood and nerve supply: (**a**) showing arterial anastomoses; (**b**) arterial supply from hand to digits (radio-opaque dye seen in arteries); (**c**) major digital arteries and nerve supply.

Nail dynamics

Clinicians used to observing the slow rate of clearance of diseased or damaged nails are apt to view the nail apparatus as a rather inert structure, although it is in fact the centre of very marked kinetic and biochemical activity.

Cell kinetics

Unlike the hair matrix, which undergoes a resting or quiescent (telogen) phase every few years, the nail matrix germinative layers continue to undertake DNA synthesis, to divide and to differentiate throughout life, akin to the epidermis in this respect. Exactly

> **The nail continues to grow unabated throughout life**

which parts of the nail apparatus contribute to the nail plate has been debated; it is now usually accepted that the three-layer nail plate is produced from the proximal matrix, the distal matrix and the nail bed (sterile ventral matrix).

Why the nail grows flat, rather than as a heaped up keratinous mass, has generated much thought and discussion. Several factors probably combine to produce a relatively flat nail plate; the orientation of the matrix rete pegs and papillae, the direction of cell differentiation and the fact that since keratinization takes place within the confines of the nail base, limited by the proximal nail fold dorsally and the terminal phalanx ventrally, the differentiating cells can only move distally and form a flat structure – by the time they leave the confines of the proximal nail fold all the cells are hardened and keratinized.

Linear nail growth

Over the last century, very many studies have been carried out on the linear growth of the nail plate in health and disease; these have been well reviewed and are listed in Tables 1.1 and 1.2. Finger nails grow at approximately 1 cm per three months and toe nails at one half of this rate.

The nails in childhood and old age

Childhood

In early childhood, the nail plate is relatively thin and may show temporary koilonychia:

Table 1.1   **Physiological and environmental factors affecting the rate of nail growth**

Faster	Slower
Daytime	Night
Pregnancy	First day of life
Minor trauma/nail biting	
Right hand nails	Left hand nails
Youth, increasing age	Old age
Fingers	Toes
Summer	Winter or cold environment
Middle, ring and index	Thumb and little
Male (?)	Female (?)

because of the shape of the matrix, some children show ridges which start laterally by the proximal nail fold and join at a central point just short of the free margin, i.e. a herringbone arrangement of the ridges. In one study 92% of normal infants between 8 and 9 weeks of age showed a single transverse line (Beau's line) on the finger nails. One child demonstrated a transverse depression through the whole nail thickness on all 20 digits.

Old age

Many of the changes seen in old age may occur in younger age groups with impaired arterial blood supply. Elastic tissue changes diffusely affecting the nail bed epidermis are often seen histologically; these changes may be due to the effects of UV radiation, although it has been stated that the nail plate is an efficient filter of UVB radiation. The whole subungual area in old age may show thickening of blood vessel walls with vascu-

Table 1.2   Pathological factors affecting the rate of nail growth

Faster	Slower
Psoriasis	Finger immobilization
normal nails	Fever
pitting	Beau's lines
onycholysis	Denervation
Pityriasis rubra pilaris	Poor nutrition
Idiopathic onycholysis of women	Kwashiorkor
Bullous ichthyosiform erythroderma	Hypothyroidism
Hyperthyroidism	Yellow nail syndrome
Drugs	Relapsing polychondritis
Arteriovenous shunts	

lar elastic tissue fragmentation. Pertinax bodies are often seen in the nail plate; they are probably remnants of nuclei of keratinocytes. Nail growth is inversely proportional to age; related to this slower growth, corneocytes are larger in old age.

The nail plate becomes paler, dull and opaque with advancing years and white nails similar to those seen in cirrhosis, uraemia and hypoalbuminaemia may be seen in normal subjects. Longitudinal ridging is present to some degree in most people after 50 years of age and this may give a 'sausage links' appearance.

For details of the common traumatic abnormalities and changes due to inadequate pedicure or neglect, detailed texts should be consulted.

Foot function

When considering toe nail problems, it is of great importance to take a full view of the

> **Always assess toe and foot shape and function when dealing with any toe nail dystrophy**

whole foot. All too often, practitioners treat the nail and foot as static anatomical structures when common problems arise as a result of their dynamic functions. When possible external and locomotor precursors of nail disease are considered, the distinct differences between finger nails and toe nails need to be taken into account. Being an appendage to the foot, the nail is often contained in footwear for long periods of time and may be subjected to the forces generated during normal locomotion. Detective work is often needed to highlight causative factors of toe nail pathology. These include:

1   Foot function
2   Foot shape
3   Footwear
4   Occupation and other factors

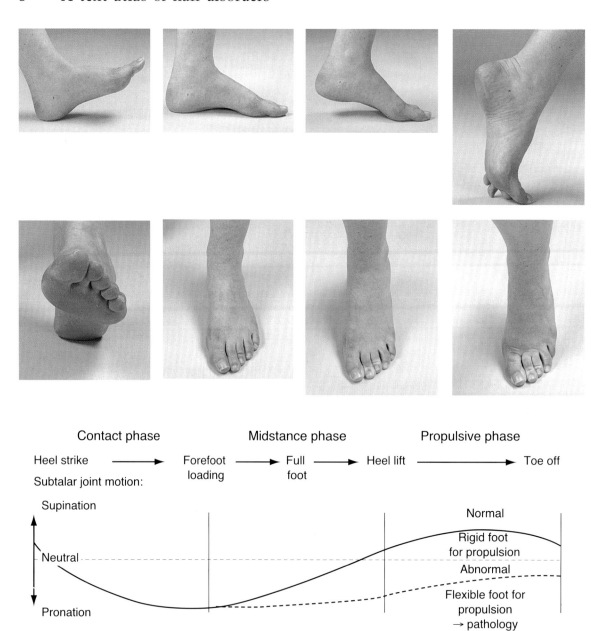

Figure 1.3

The positions of the foot during the normal gait cycle.

In simple terms, the human foot has evolved to carry out a specific function – to assist smooth and efficient locomotion. In undertaking this task the foot has developed the ability to alter its structure and, as a consequence, its function within a single footstep. To understand this we must briefly look at the normal gait cycle (Figure 1.3). During normal walking, the first stage (heel strike) begins when the heel comes into contact with the ground. To permit shock absorption the foot must become a flexible unit. It does this by pronation (a triplanar movement occurring mainly at the subtalar and midtarsal joints of the foot). It may be recognized by eversion of the calcaneum, lowering of the arch and slight elongation in the foot length. Subtalar joint pronation unlocks the midtarsal joint so that effectively the foot is flexible to accommodate ground reaction at heel strike. This pronation continues until the whole of the foot is flat to the floor (midstance or full foot). In order for this foot to take full body weight as the opposite foot leaves the ground, it must now become a rigid unit. Once the other limb has passed the plantigrade foot, and undergoes heel strike, the foot begins propulsion – the heel lifts, so body weight is shifted onto the forefoot and the toes. In order to stabilize the foot and balance the whole body forward, the foot becomes supinated. (This is a movement involving the subtalar and midtarsal joints whereby the calcaneum inverts, the arch is raised and the foot is shortened.) This movement effectively locks the foot into rigidity allowing a stable platform for propulsion.

Many abnormal foot functions can upset this sequence of supination–pronation–resupination. In terms of toe nail pathology, these primarily occur around the propulsive phase of the gait cycle. If for any reason the foot has been unable to supinate to an adequate degree, there may not be adequate rigidity and propulsion occurs on a 'flexible' foot. So major forces may be dissipated through the forefoot. When repeated many hundreds of times a day, this can have adverse effects on the digital area, especially when interacting with footwear. If a foot is pronating excessively on propulsion, the foot will elongate (as part pronation) so the distal area will be subject to trauma if the footwear is inadequate in length. Control of the excessive pronation may be obtained by way of prescribed orthoses in footwear.

Foot shape

Foot shape is also of major importance when considering precursors to toe nail disease. Within any population there is great variation in foot shape and it is important to bear in mind that foot shape will change with age and the effects of disease. A good example is hallux valgus (Figure 1.4, Figure 1.5): at a young age all that may be apparent is slight first metatarsal head enlargement, but within a few years one sees the gradual deviation of the hallux laterally, often underriding the second toe and forcing it into the upper of a shoe. Such changes in foot shape will inevitably affect foot and nail function. Commonly, medial rotation of the toe accompanied by its abduction towards the second toe causes the flesh around the nail edge to roll over the nail plate – a precursor to the development of ingrowing toe nails.

Hallux rigidus is a common condition in which there is a reduction in the normal range of motion at the first metatarsophalangeal joint. It is characterized by an enlargement of the metatarsal head and a general stiffening of the joint; motion is obtained at the nearest functional joint – the interphalangeal joint of the hallux. Over time, this leads to a fixed dorsiflexed distal phalanx; the nail often protrudes dorsally and is open to trauma from footwear and stubbing.

Problems with the lesser digits can also adversely affect the nail apparatus (Figures 1.6–1.10); these can be congenital or acquired. Commonly seen is the foot with the second toe slightly longer than the first (Figure 1.10). This can lead to the longer toe suffering increased trauma from the end of a shoe or stubbing and secondary onychomycosis. Longer toes may suffer trauma in the shoe leading to subungual haematoma and consequent long-term changes in the nail structure. Other types of digital deformities may also predispose to pathology of the nail. Neurological disturbances within the lower limb as a result of diabetes, paresis or other disorders can lead to changes in muscular tone within the leg. Spasticity or atrophy may lead to imbalances between dorsiflexors or plantarflexors of the foot which, in turn, result in digital deformities and nail distortion; the latter will vary in relation to the specific paralysis or orthopaedic change.

Footwear

Footwear is most often overlooked as a causative or contributory factor in nail

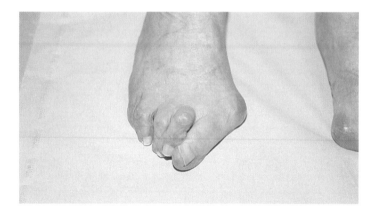

Figure 1.4

Hallux abductovalgus.

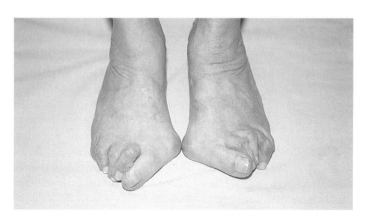

Figure 1.5

Hallux abductovalgus. Rotation of the digit can place extra pressure around the nail when walking.

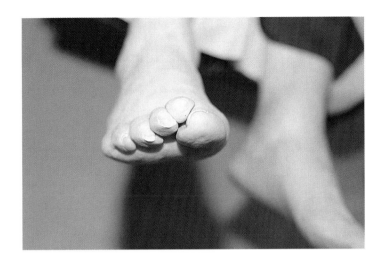

Figure 1.6

Overlapping toes can lead to nail deformity long term. Note early involution, lateral sulcus of hallux.

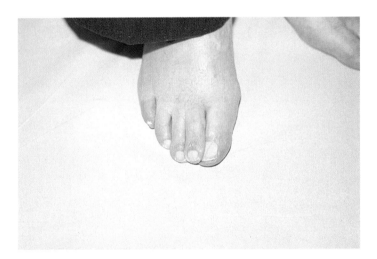

Figure 1.7

Same foot as Figure 1.6 – weight bearing.

> **Most toe nail dystrophies are modified by footwear and foot wear!**

disease. When questioned about their footwear, patients will often state that their shoes feel comfortable: 'it's just my toe nail that hurts when I wear them'. Nail pathology from shoes can be due to many factors:

- Poor fitting of footwear.
- Inadequate footwear design or construction.
- Excessive wear to shoes.

When looking at shoe fitting, areas of prime importance are:

- Heel height – generally if heels are too high, the foot is forced forward into the

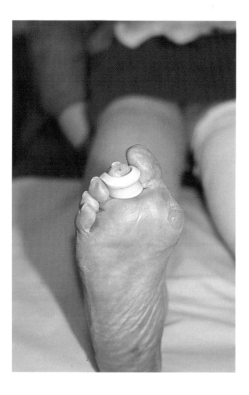

Figure 1.8

Silicon toe prop – designed to prevent apical weight bearing in deformed toes.

toe box with every step, traumatizing the anterior part of the foot, especially around the nail apparatus and apices. The higher the heel, the more damage is likely to occur. It has been the experience of the authors that heel heights greater than 30–35 mm can yield unwanted effects.

- Lack of a suitable fastening – a foot in a shoe without adequate fastening suffers in that the foot is free to move unrestrained in the shoe and inevitably (as with high heels) it tends to slip forward into the toe box region of the shoe, traumatizing the distal aspect. Laces are, by far, the best method of fastening in a shoe and the higher the laces come up from the front of the shoe the more restraint and support is given to the foot. With patients who, due to arthritic fingers or spine, cannot tie laces, velcro straps make a reasonable substitute (Figure 1.11).

- Poor toe box design – in order to restrict rubbing and other trauma to the forefoot and nails, a good toe box is a vital feature. Adequate depth and width ensure that no undue pressure is placed on the digital

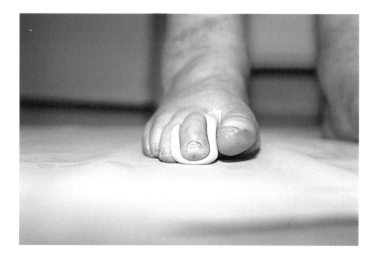

Figure 1.9

Silicon toe prop – same as in Figure 1.8 – weight bearing.

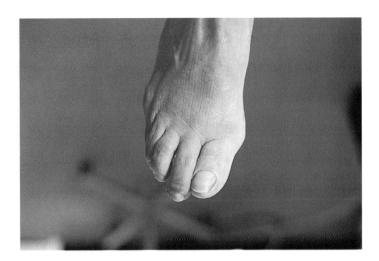

Figure 1.10

Long second toe – nail may be selectively subjected to traumatic factors.

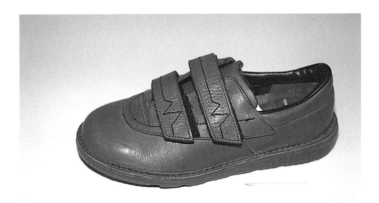

Figure 1.11

Shoe with velcro straps (alternative to lace ups).

areas (Figure 1.12); allied with a suitable fastening, this ensures that the foot stays well back from the tip of the shoe and into the heel. In modern shoes, manufacturers still produce types with inadequate width and depth in the toe box area. One can often see the effects of this when toe outlines are visible from the outside of the shoe. When looking at toe nail problems it is wise to feel inside the upper of the shoe; one may often feel a dent or tear in the inner lining of the shoe corresponding to the affected digit. Other clues can be given by the nail itself. A nail with unusual pigmentation may have acquired this from rubbing on the leather of new shoes. More commonly though, a single toe nail with a very 'polished' sheen to it can be the result of continuous rubbing on the soft lining of an upper of a shoe.

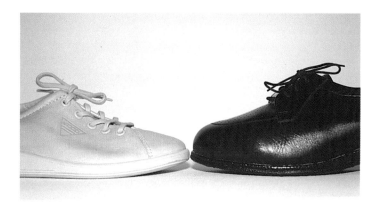

Figure 1.12

Shoes positioned tip to tip, highlighting different depths as a possible contribution to nail problems.

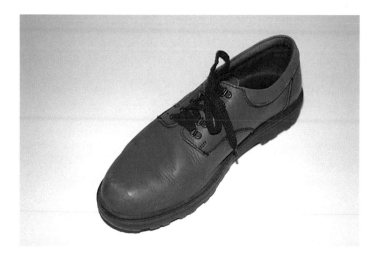

Figure 1.13

Shoe with a seamless front – a good design feature to prevent trauma to digits.

- Seams which run over the toe box region of the shoe to give an aesthetic touch can be a cause of problems. Inside the shoe the stitching producing the seam may be readily felt in the shoe upper, impinging on the toe area; such stitching is best avoided (Figure 1.13).
- Shoes which are too long or without a fastening can often lead to increased nail trauma as, to compensate for the excessive movement, toes become clawed to maintain ground contact and increase stability. Whether poor fitting shoes are a direct cause of digital deformity continues to be debated.

Specially made shoes for specific foot cum toe disorders may be invaluable. For example, the use of half shoes in conjunction with standard diabetic foot care substantially improves outpatient treatment of neuropathic foot/toe ulcers and may be of great help in painful periungual changes.

Occupational and other factors

When looking at causative factors of nail problems one must always take into account patients' circumstances. The amount of time a person spends on their feet may affect the severity of the nail problem. Moreover, the footwear worn for these periods of time will be crucial. Occupational footwear can be notorious for precipitating such problems.

Occlusive type footwear worn for long periods of time can lead to retention of excessive perspiration. This may predispose to infection which may go on to affect the nail and surrounding tissues. This is often seen in manual workers who spend long periods of time in rubber or plastic boots or similar footwear.

The transportation and construction industries provide the highest incidence of foot injuries. Since the introduction of steel toe cap shoes the incidence has been reduced, but even these are not without their problems. The rigidity of the toe box has meant that incorrectly fitting boots have led to toe and nail injuries as a result of their design.

In conclusion, the way in which the foot functions and interacts with footwear may have a detrimental effect on the health of the nail, its surrounding structures and any diseases that occur due to other primary causes.

2 Nail configuration abnormalities

Clubbing (Hippocratic fingers)

The bulbous digital deformity known as clubbing (Figures 2.1a, b) was described as early as the fifth century BC when Hippocrates noted such changes in patients suffering from empyema. The diagnostic signs comprise:

1   Overcurvature of the nails in the proximal to distal and transverse planes (Figure 2.2)
2   Enlargement of periungual soft tissue structures confined to the tip of each digit

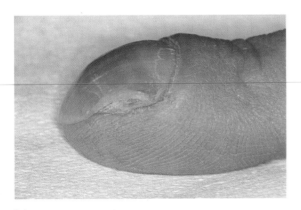

(a)

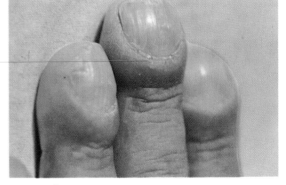

(b)

Figure 2.1

(a,b) Clubbing.

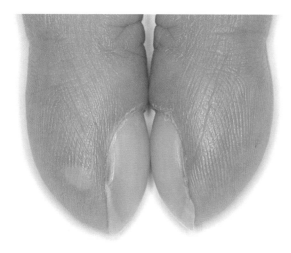

Figure 2.2

Clubbing – demonstrating typical nail curvature.

The increased nail curvature usually affects all 20 digits, but may be particularly obvious on the thumbs, index and middle fingers. The 'watch-glass' deformity of the nail may occur as an isolated deformity without any associated enlargement of the tip of the digit. The shape of the curved nails is variable and may appear fusiform, like a bird's beak, or clubbed like a watch-glass. The matrix quite often appears abnormally large.

There are three main types of clubbing:

1   Simple type.
2   Hypertrophic pulmonary osteoarthropathy.
3   Pachydermoperiostosis.

The simple type

This is the most common category and has several distinctive characteristics:

1   Increased nail curvature with a transverse furrow separating it from the rest of the nail both in the early stage and after resolution. The onset is usually gradual and painless, except in some cases of carcinoma of the lung in which clubbing may develop abruptly and be associated with severe pain.
2   Hypertrophy of the soft parts of the terminal segment due to firm, elastic, oedematous infiltration of the pulp, which may spread on to the dorsal surface with marked periungual swelling.
3   Hyperplasia of the dermal fibrovascular tissue which may extend to involve the adjacent matrix. This accounts for one of the earliest signs of clubbing – abnormal mobility of the nail base which can be rocked back and forth giving the impression that it is floating on a soft oedematous pad. The increased vascularity is responsible for the slow return of colour when the nail is pressed and released.
4   Acral cyanosis is often observed.

In the early stages clubbing may involve one hand only, though eventually both hands become affected symmetrically. Several stages of clubbing or acropachy may be distinguished: suspected, slight, average and severe. In practice the degree of the deformity may be gauged by Lovibond's `profile sign' which measures the angle between the curved nail plate and the proximal nail fold when the finger is viewed from the radial aspect. This is normally 160°, but exceeds 180° in clubbing. With a modified profile sign one measures the angle between the middle and the terminal phalanx at the interphalangeal joint. In normal fingers the distal phalanx forms an almost straight (180°) extension of the middle phalanx, whereas in severe clubbing this angle may be reduced to 160° or even 140°. However, the best indicator may well be the simple clinical method adopted by Schamroth: in normal individuals a distinct aperture or 'window', usually diamond-shaped, is formed at the base of the nail bed; early clubbing obliterates this window.

Radiological changes occur in less than one-fifth of cases. These include phalangeal demineralization and irregular thickening of the cortical diaphysis. Ungual tufts generally show considerable variations and may be very prominent in advanced stages of the disease. Bony atrophy may be present.

Congenital finger clubbing may be accompanied by changes such as hyperkeratosis of the palms and soles, and cortical hypertrophy of the long bones. Familial clubbing may be associated with hypertrophic osteoarthropathy; some authors regard simple clubbing as a mild form of the latter. Isolated watch-glass nails without other deformities are also constitutionally determined.

Very rare cases of unilateral Hippocratic nails have been reported due to obstructed circulation, oedema of the soft tissues and dystrophy of the affected parts. The pathological process apparently responsible for clubbing and its associated changes is the increased blood flow due to the opening of many anastomotic shunts.

> **Acquired clubbing almost always has an internal cause**

Hypertrophic pulmonary osteoarthropathy

This disorder is characterized by the following five signs:

1 Clubbing of the nails.
2 Hypertrophy of the upper and lower extremities similar to the deformity found in acromegaly.
3 Joint changes with pseudo-inflammatory, symmetrical, painful arthropathy of the large limb joints, especially those of the legs. This syndrome is almost pathognomonic of malignant chest tumours, especially lung carcinoma and mesothelioma of the pleura; less commonly bronchiectasis is seen. Gynaecomastia may also be present.
4 There may be bone changes such as bilateral, proliferative periostitis and moderate, diffuse decalcification.
5 Peripheral neurovascular disorders such as local cyanosis and paraesthesia are not uncommon.

Hypertrophic osteoarthropathy confined to the lower extremities appears as a manifestation of arterial graft sepsis.

Pachydermoperiostosis

Pachydermoperiostosis (idiopathic hypertrophic osteoarthropathy) is very rare. In most of the reported cases the digital changes typically begin at or about the time of puberty. The ends of the fingers and toes are bulbous and often grotesquely shaped, with hyperhidrosis of the hands and the feet (Figure 2.3). The clubbing stops abruptly at the distal interphalangeal joint. In this type the lesions of the fingertips are clinically identical to those of hypertrophic pulmonary osteoarthropathy. However, in pachydermoperiostosis, the thickened cortex appears

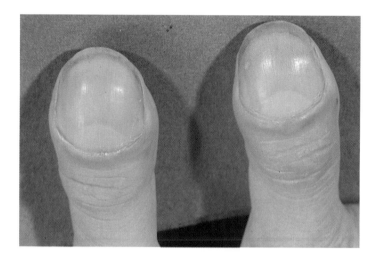

Figure 2.3

Clubbing – pachydermoperiostosis.

homogeneous on X-ray examination and does not impinge on the medullary space. Acroosteolysis of the distal phalanges has been reported.

The pachydermal change of the extremities and face, with furrowing and oiliness of the skin, is the most characteristic feature of the disorder; it is described in the French literature as the Touraine, Solente and Golé syndrome. Nevertheless, in hypertrophic pulmonary osteo-arthropathy there may be facial skin and scalp changes which are indistinguishable from those seen in pachydermoperiostosis; this may be due to a common genetic factor. In the differential diagnosis acromegaly must be considered; this enhances tufting of the terminal phalanges and presents an 'anchor-like' appearance, but without acro-osteolysis. Thyroid acropachy is usually associated with exophthalmus, pretibial myxoedema and abnormal thyroid function.

It should be noted that only rarely will any type of clubbing present to a dermatologist, since in most cases it is simply one sign among many relating to the primary cause.

Comprehensive classification of clubbing

The principal general causes of clubbing are shown in Table 2.1; a comprehensive list of causes follows.

Idiopathic forms

Hereditary and congenital forms sometimes associated with other anomalies:

* Familial and genotypic pachydermoperiostosis
* Racial forms (Negroid individuals; North Africans)
* Syndrome of pernio, periostosis and lipodystrophy
* Muckle–Wells syndrome

Table 2.1   General causes of clubbing and pseudoclubbing

Clubbing

Unilateral	Aortic/subclavian aneurysm
	Brachial plexus injury
	Trauma (Figure 2.4)
Lower extremity	Arterial graft sepsis
General	
Congenital	Familial/sporadic
Thoracic tumours (bronchopulmonary cancers)	
Pulmonary	
Cardiovascular	
Gastrointestinal	Inflammatory bowel disease
	Parasitosis
	Liver disease
	Tropical sprue
Endocrine/metabolic	Thyroid, acromegaly (Figure 2.5)
	Malnutrition
AIDS	Secondary to pulmonary and other infections; hashish, heroin (upper extremities)
Pseudoclubbing	Yellow nail syndrome (Figure 2.6)
	Gout
	Sarcoidosis
	Osteoid osteoma
	Metastases
	Congenital abnormalities
	Chronic paronychia – severe hook nail

Acquired forms

1 Thoracic disorders
These are involved in about 80% of cases of clubbing, often with the common denominator of hypoxia:
  • Broncho-pulmonary diseases, especially chronic and infective bronchiectasis, abscess and cyst of the lung, pulmonary tuberculosis
  • Sarcoidosis, pulmonary fibrosis, emphysema, Ayerza's syndrome, chronic pulmonary venous engorgement, asthma in infancy, mucoviscidosis
  • Blastomycosis, pneumonia, pneumocystis carinii, AIDS

2 Thoracic tumours:
  • Primary or metastatic bronchopulmonary cancers, pleural tumours, mediastinal tumours
  • Hodgkin's disease, lymphoma, pseudotumour due to oesophageal dilatation

3 Cardiovascular diseases:
  • Congenital heart disease associated with cyanosis (rarely non-cyanotic)

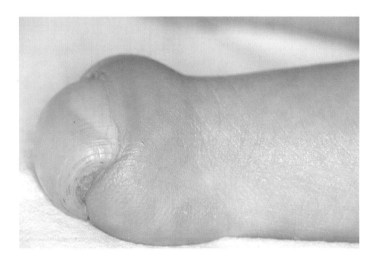

Figure 2.4

Pseudoclubbing due to trauma – hooked nail deformity.

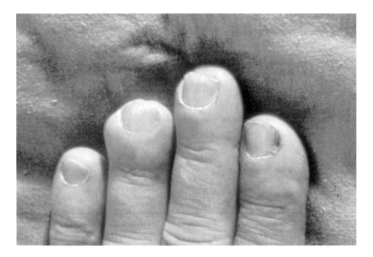

Figure 2.5

Clubbed appearance in acromegaly. (Courtesy of D. Wendling.)

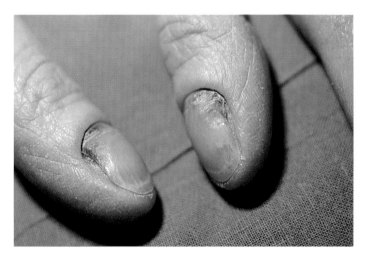

Figure 2.6

Pseudoclubbing in yellow nail syndrome.

- Thoracic vascular malformations; stenoses and arteriovenous aneurysms
- Osler's disease (subacute bacterial endocarditis)
- Congestive cardiac failure
- Myxoma
- Raynaud's syndrome, erythromelalgia, Maffucci's syndrome

4 Disorders of the alimentary tract
These are involved in 5% of cases:
- Oesophageal, gastric and colonic cancer
- Diseases of the small intestine
- Colonic diseases
- Amoebiasis and inflammatory states of the colon
- Ulcerative colitis
- Familial polyposis, Gardner's syndrome
- Ascariasis
- Active chronic hepatitis
- Primary or secondary cirrhoses
- Purgative abuse

5 Endocrine origin:
- Diamond's syndrome (pretibial myxoedema, exophthalmus and finger clubbing)
- Acromegaly

6 Haematological causes:
- Methaemoglobinemia
- Sulphaemoglobinemia
- Haemoglobinopathies
- Primary polycythaemia or secondary polycythaemia associated with hypoxia
- Poisoning by phosphorus, arsenic, alcohol, mercury or beryllium

7 Hypervitaminosis A
8 Malnutrition, kwashiorkor
9 Addiction (hashish, heroin)
10 Syringomyelia, POEM syndrome
11 Lupus erythematosus
12 Unilateral or limited to a few digits:
- Subluxation of the shoulder (with paralysis of the brachial plexus), medial nerve neuritis

- Pancoast–Tobias' syndrome
- Aneurysm of the aorta or the subclavian artery
- Sarcoidosis
- Tophaceous gout

13 Lower extremities:
- Arterial graft sepsis

14 Isolated forms:
- Local injury, whitlow, lymphangitis
- Subungual epidermoid inclusions

15 Transitory form:
- Physiological in the newborn child (due to reversal of the circulation at birth)

16 Occupational acro-osteolysis (exposure to vinyl chloride)

Koilonychia (spoon-shaped nails)

Koilonychia is more often due to local rather than systemic factors

This sign is the opposite of clubbing. The nail is firmly attached to bone by vertical dermal connective tissue bundles in the subungual area which bond directly to the bony periosteum.

In the early stages of koilonychia there is flattening of the nail plate. Later, the edges become everted upwards and the nail appears concave, thus the descriptive term 'spoon nail' (Figures 2.7, 2.8, 2.9). In mild cases the water test may enable a drop of water to be retained on the nail plate. The subungual tissues may be normal, or affected by hyperkeratosis at the lateral and/or the distal margin.

The main types of koilonychia are:

- In neonates and in infancy, koilonychia is a temporary physiological condition

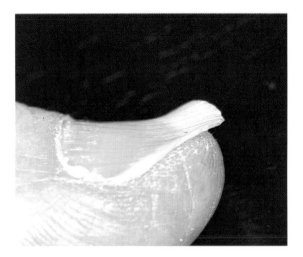

Figure 2.7

Koilonychia – 'spoon-shaped' nail; thin nail variety.

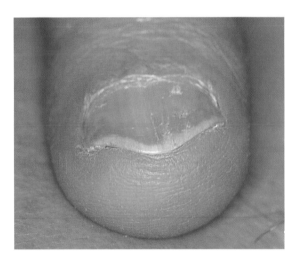

Figure 2.8

Koilonychia – distal view with some terminal traumatic whitening.

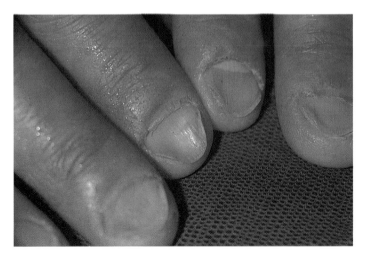

Figure 2.9

Koilonychia – severe variety, of many nails.

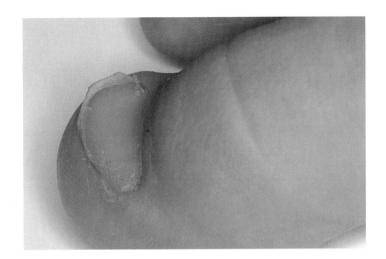

Figure 2.10

Koilonychia – temporary type of early infancy.

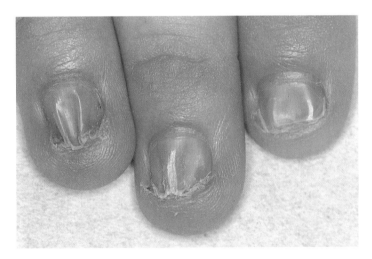

Figure 2.11

Koilonychia in hereditary ectodermal dysplasia.

(Figure 2.10). There is a proven correlation between koilonychia and iron deficiency (with normal haemoglobin values) in infants.

- Koilonychia is a common manifestation of the rare Plummer–Vinson syndrome in association with anaemia, dysphagia and glossitis.

When subungual keratosis accompanies koilonychia, psoriasis should be considered, as well as occupational causes, which may be relevant in those who work with cement, or in car mechanics whose hands suffer constant immersion in oil, for example.

- Thin nails of any cause (old age, peripheral arterial disease and so on).
- Soft nails of any cause (mainly occupational).
- Hereditary and congenital forms (Figure 2.11), sometimes associated with other nail signs such as leukonychia.

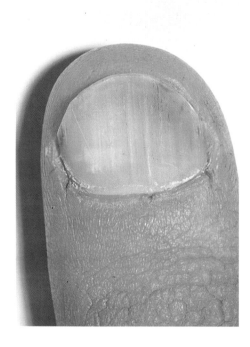

Figure 2.12

Koilonychia – transverse and longitudinal curvature evident.

Table 2.2   Commonest causes of koilonychia

Physiological	Early childhood (Figure 2.10)
Idiopathic	
Congenital	LEOPARD syndrome
	Ectodermal dysplasias (Figure 2.11)
	Trichothiodystrophy
	Nail–patella syndrome
Acquired	
Metabolic/endocrine	Iron deficiency
	Acromegaly
	Haemochromatosis
	Porphyria
	Renal dialysis/transplant
	Thyroid disease
Dermatoses	Alopecia areata
	Darier's disease
	Lichen planus
	Psoriasis
	Raynaud's syndrome
Occupational	Contact with oils, e.g. engineering industry
Infections	Onychomycosis
	Syphilis
Traumatic	Toes of rickshaw boys
Carpal tunnel syndrome	

The commonest causes of koilonychia are probably occupational softening (Figure 2.12) and iron deficiency. Table 2.2 lists most of the well known causes.

Transverse overcurvature

There are three main types of this condition: the arched, pincer or trumpet nail; the tile-shaped nail; and a third less common variety, the 'plicatured' nail (Figure 2.13). Table 2.3 lists some of the causes of transverse overcurvature.

> **Transverse overcurvature may cause ingrowing nail of the hand**

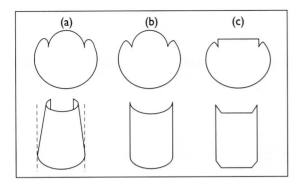

Figure 2.13

Transverse overcurvature showing the three sub-types: **(a)** pincer or trumpet nail; **(b)** tile-shaped nail; and **(c)** plicatured nail with sharply angled lateral margins.

Table 2.3   **Commonest causes of transverse overcurvature**

Congenital
Hidrotic ectodermal dysplasia
Hypohidrotic ectodermal dysplasia
Congenital onychodysplasia of index finger nails
Yellow nail syndrome (Figure 2.15)
Pseudo yellow nail syndrome (insecticides and weed killers) (Figure 2.16)

Developmental
Pincer nails (*see* Figures 2.14a, 2.15)

Acquired
Osteoarthritis (see Figures 2.14b, 2.14d)
Neglect, e.g. of toe nails in old age

Pincer nail

Pincer nail is characterized by transverse overcurvature that increases along the longitudinal axis of the nail and reaches its greatest proportion towards the tip (Figures 2.14a–d). At this point, the lateral borders tighten around the soft tissues which are pinched without necessarily disrupting the epidermis. Eventually the soft tissue may actually disappear, sometimes accompanied by resorption of the underlying bone. Subungual exostosis may present in this way: the dorsal extension of bone producing the pincer nail; the exostosis must be excised. The lateral borders of the nail exert a constant pressure, permanently constricting the deformed nail plate (unguis constringens). In extreme cases, they may join together, forming a tunnel; or they may become rolled taking the form of a cone. In certain varieties, the nails are shaped like claws, resembling pachyonychia congenita.

This morphological abnormality would be no more than a curiosity if the constriction were not occasionally accompanied by pain which can be provoked by the lightest of touch, such as the weight of a bedsheet. There are a number of subtypes of this condition:

1   The inherited form, usually showing symmetrical involvement both of the great toe nails and of the lesser toe nails. The great toe nails typically have lateral deviation of their longitudinal axis, the lesser toe nails being deviated medially. This dystrophy is a developmental abnormality which may be an autosomal dominant trait. The pathogenesis of the nail plate deformation has recently been clarified: the great toe nail, which is normally curved transversally, spreads around almost 40% of the dorsal aspect of the base of the terminal phalanx. Radiographs demonstrate that in subjects with pincer nails the base of the terminal

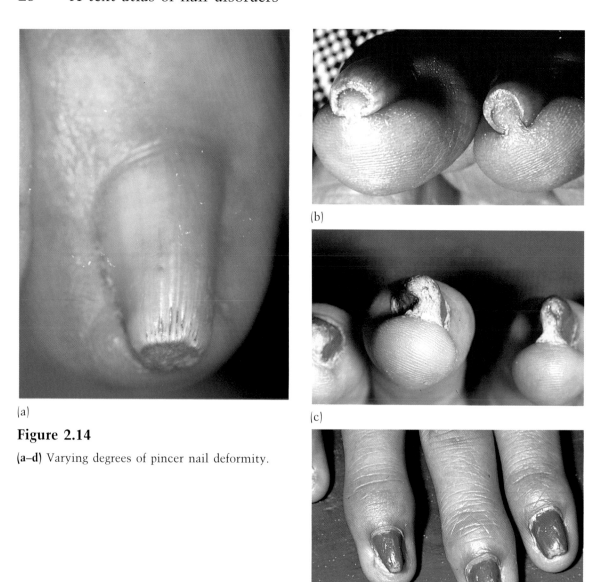

(a)

(b)

(c)

(d)

Figure 2.14

(a–d) Varying degrees of pincer nail deformity.

phalanx is widened by lateral osteophytes that are even more pronounced on the medial aspect of the phalanx. By widening the transverse curvature of the nail at its proximal end it becomes more curved distally. This can easily be shown by trying to flatten a curved elastic sheet at one end: the other end will increase its

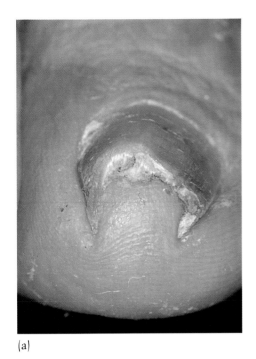

(a)

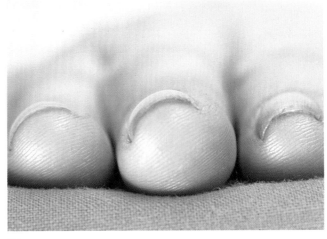

(b)

Figure 2.15

(a) Transverse curvature of nail; (b) transverse curvature of nail in yellow syndrome (before colour change).

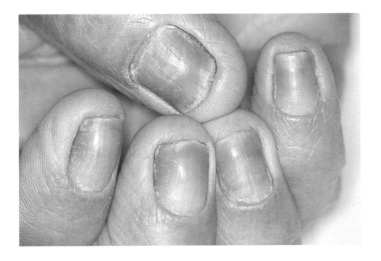

Figure 2.16

Transverse overcurvature in the pseudo yellow nail syndrome due to insecticide.

curve. The asymmetry of the lateral osteophytes explains why the lateral deviation of the nail is even more pronounced than that of the distal phalanx.

2   Other examples can be attributed to wearing ill-fitting shoes. These acquired pincer nails are not usually symmetrical and the lesser toe nails are not generally affected.

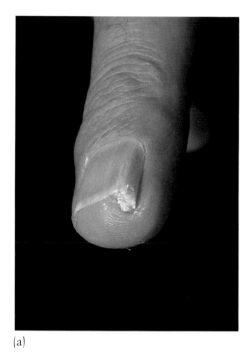

(a)

(b)

Figure 2.17

(a) Transverse overcurvature of nail: unilateral plicature; (b) transverse overcurvature of nail: bilateral plicatured variety (*see* Figure 2.13).

3 Underlying pathology, such as subungual exostosis of the toes and inflammatory osteoarthritis, should always be looked for, especially if the fingers are involved.
4 Some dermatological disorders, especially psoriasis, may also cause transverse overcurvature of the nails.

lateral margins being sharply angled forming vertical sides which are parallel (Figure 2.17a, b). Although these deformities may be associated with ingrowing nails, inflammatory oedema due to the constriction of the enclosed soft tissues is unusual.

Tile-shaped nail

The tile-shaped nail presents with an increase in the transverse curvature; the lateral edges of the nail remain parallel.

Plicatured nail

In the plicatured variety the surface of the nail plate is almost flat, with one or both

Dolichonychia (long nails)

In this condition the length of the nail is much greater than the width (Figure 2.18). It has been described in:

1 Ehlers Danlos syndrome
2 Marfan's syndrome (Figure 2.19)
3 Eunuchoidism
4 Hypopituitarism
5 Hypohidrotic ectodermal dysplasia

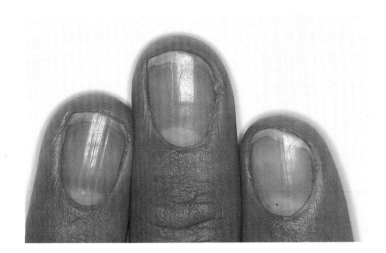

Figure 2.18

Dolichonychia – long nails.

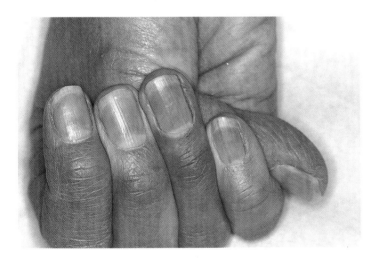

Figure 2.19

Dolichonychia – Marfan's syndrome.

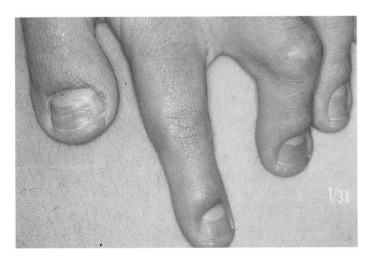

Figure 2.20

Brachyonychia – Rubinstein–Taybi type, broad thumb. (Courtesy of P. Souteyrand.)

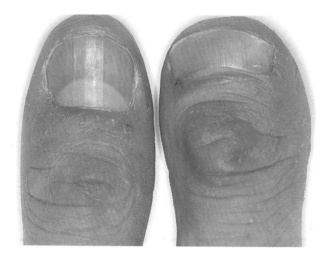

Figure 2.21
Brachyonychia – short nail.

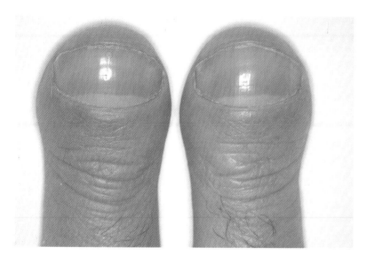

Figure 2.22
Bilateral brachyonychia – racquet
nail associated with clubbing.
(Courtesy of F. David, Paris)

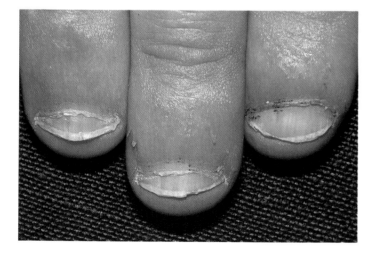

Figure 2.23
Brachyonychia – severe variant.

Brachyonychia (short nails)

In this condition, the width of the nail plate (and the nail bed) is greater than the length. It may occur in isolation or in association with shortening of the terminal phalanx. This 'racquet thumb' is usually inherited as an autosomal dominant trait. All the fingers may rarely be involved. The epiphyses of the terminal phalanx of the thumb usually undergo closure between 13 and 14 years of age in girls, slightly later in boys. In individuals with this hereditary defect the epiphyseal line is obliterated on the affected side by 7 to 10 years of age, only occurring at the usual later age in the normal thumb. Since periosteal growth continues, the result is a deformed, racquet-like thumb.

Racquet nails have been reported in association with brachydactylia and multiple malignant Spiegler tumours. A syndrome of broad thumbs, broad great toes, facial abnormalities and mental retardation has also been described. Table 2.4 lists many well recognized causes of short nails, whilst Table 2.5 gives details of the rarer hereditary and congenital conditions in which it can occur.

Table 2.4 **Causes of brachyonychia**

Congenital
Rubenstein–Taybi: 'broad thumbs' syndrome (Figure 2.20)
Micronychia with trisomy 21
Congenital malalignment – great toe nails

Acquired
Isolated defect: racquet thumb (Figures 2.21–2.23) (in fact hereditary)
Nail biters (Figure 2.24)
Associated with bone resorption in hyperparathyroidism (Figure 2.25)
Psoriatic arthropathy (Figure 2.26)

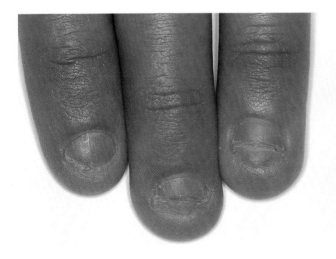

Figure 2.24
Brachyonychia – nail biting.

Table 2.5 Hereditary forms of broad nails (some also with pseudoclubbing)

Disease	Inheritance	Clinical features
Acrocephalosyndactyly	AD	Craniosynostosis, syndactyly, ankylosis and other skeletal deformities.
Acrodysostosis	AD	Finger nails short, broad and oval in shape. Short fingers. Nasal and midface hypoplasia. Mental retardation. Growth failure. Pigmented naevi.
Berk–Tabatznik syndrome	?	Stub thumb, short terminal phalanges of all fingers except digit V. Bilateral optic atrophy, cervical kyphosis.
Familial mandibuloacral dysplasia	AR	Club-shaped terminal phalanges. Mandibular hypoplasia, delayed cranial closure. Dysplastic clavicles. Atrophy of skin over hands and feet. Alopecia.
Keipert syndrome	AR or XR	Unusual facies with large nose. Protruded upper lip. Short and broad distal phalanges of halluces and fingers, except digit V.
Larsen's syndrome	AR or AD	Stub thumbs, cylindrical fingers. Flattened peculiar facies, widespread eyes. Multiple dislocations, short metacarpals.
Nanocephalic dwarfism	AR	Low birth weight with adult head circumference. Mental retardation. Beak-like protrusion of nose. Multiple osseous anomalies. Clubbing of fingers.
Otopalatodigital syndrome	XR or AR	Broad, short nails, especially of thumbs and big toes. Mental retardation. Prominent occiput. Hypoplasia of facial bones. Cloven palate. Conductive deafness.
Pleonosteosis	?	Short stature. Spade-like thumbs with thick palmar pads. Massive, 'knobby' thumbs. Short flexed fingers. Limited joint motion with contractures.
Pseudohypoparathyroidism	XD or AR	Short stature. Round face. Depressed nasal bridge. Short metacarpals. Mental retardation. Cataracts in 25%. Enamel hypoplasia. Calcifications in skin.
Puretic syndrome	?	Osteolysis of peripheral phalanges. Stunted growth. Contracture of joints. Multiple subcutaneous nodules. Atrophic sclerodermic skin.
Rubinstein–Taybi syndrome	AD	Broad thumb with radial angulation and great toes. High palate. Short stature. Mental retardation. Peculiar facies.
Spiegler tumours and racquet nails	?	Brachydactyly. Turban tumours.
Stub thumb with racquet nail (Figures 2.21, 2.22)	AD	No other defects. Appears at the age of 7 to 10 years with early obliteration of the epiphyseal line.

AD: autosomal dominant; AR: autosomal recessive; XD: sex-linked dominant; XR: sex-linked recessive.

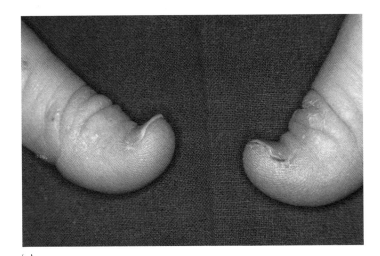

(a)

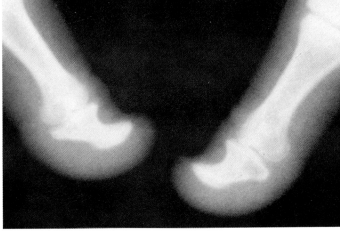

(b)

Figure 2.25

(a) Brachyonychia – associated with bone resorption in hyperpara-thyroidism; (b) radiograph of (a). (Courtesy of B. Schubert.)

Parrot beak nails

In this symmetrical overcurvature of the free edge, some finger nails mimic the beak of a parrot (Figures 2.27, 2.28); this shape disappears temporarily if the nails are soaked in lukewarm water for about 30 minutes. This is often not seen in clinical practice because such patients usually trim their nails close to the line of separation from the nail bed.

Hook and claw-like nails

One or both little toe nails are often rounded like a claw (Figures 2.29, 2.30). This condition predominates in women wearing high heels and narrow shoes and is often associated with the development of hyperkeratosis such as calluses on the feet. Congenital claw-like fingers and toe nails have been reported. Claw nails may be curved dorsally showing

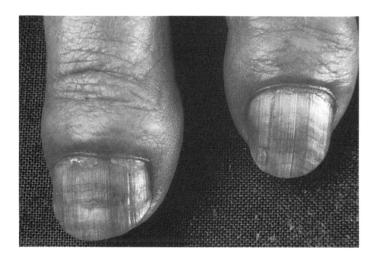

Figure 2.26

Brachyonychia – in psoriatic arthropathy. (Courtesy of P. Combemale, Lyon)

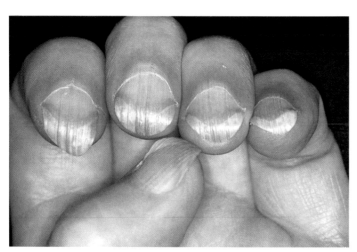

Figure 2.27

Parrot-beak nails.

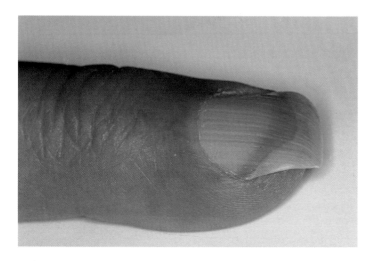

Figure 2.28

Parrot-beak nails – lateral view.

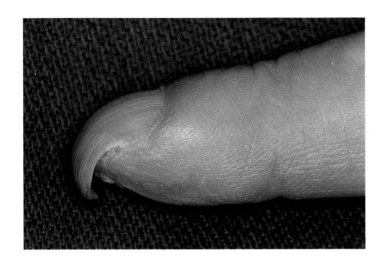

Figure 2.29

Claw-like nail.

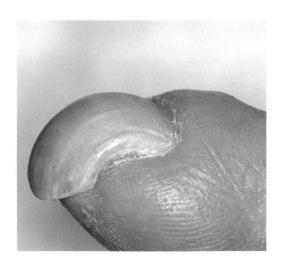

Figure 2.30

Hook nail.

a concave upper surface, resembling onycho-gryphosis or post-traumatic hook nail. In the nail–patella syndrome when the pointed lunula sign occurs, if the nail is not manicured it will tend to grow with a pointed tip, resembling a claw. Hook-shaped nails may be an isolated defect, congenital or acquired (e.g. traumatic).

Micro- and macronychia and polydactyly

In Iso Kikuchi (congenital onychodysplasia of index finger nails or COIF) syndrome there are two types of micronychia. The most frequent is medially sited; in 'rolled'

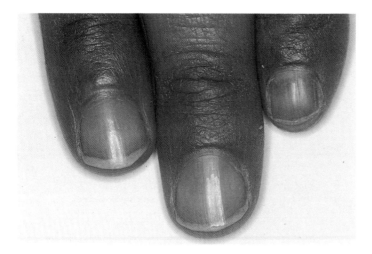

Figure 2.31

Micronychia involving one finger.

micronychia the nail is centrally located (Figures 2.31–2.33). Figures 2.34 and 2.35 illustrate other examples of congenital micronychia. Overlapping of the nail surface by an enlarged lateral nail fold may result in apparent micronychia (Turner's syndrome).

In macronychia the nails of one or more digits are wider than normal, with nail bed and matrix similarly affected (Figure 2.36). They may occur as an isolated defect or in association with megadactyly, as in von Recklinghausen's disease, epiloia and Proteus syndrome (Figure 2.37). Table 2.6 lists the known associations of micro- and macronychia.

Duplication of the thumb is a sign of congenital polydactyly, one of the commonest anomalies of the hand. The frequency of polydactyly of the hands has been estimated to be 0.37%; it is more common than polydactyly of the feet (Figure 2.38). Seven types of thumb polydactyly can be distinguished according to the level of bone bifurcation. Patients with types 1 and 2 thumb polydactyly have two distinct nails separated by a longitudinal incision or a unique nail with a central indentation of the distal margin. Symphalangism is commonly

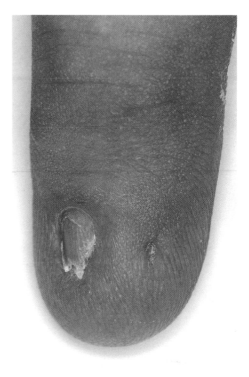

Figure 2.32

Micronychia – congenital onychodysplasia of index fingernails (COIF syndrome).

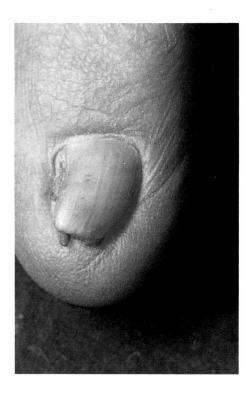

Figure 2.33

Rolled micronychia.

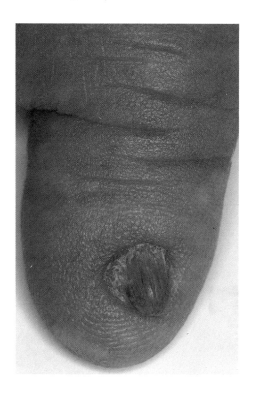

Figure 2.34

Micronychia – congenital ectodermal dysplasia.

Table 2.6   Causes of micro- and macronychia

Congenital
   Ectodermal dysplasias (Figures 2.34, 2.35)
   Congenital onchodysplasia of index finger
      nails (Figures 2.32, 2.33)
   Bifid toe (Figure 2.38)
   Dyskeratosis congenita
   Chromosomal abnormalities
   Nail–patella syndrome

Acquired
   Fetal teratogens
      Hydantoinates
      Alcohol
      Warfarin
   Amniotic bands

observed. Thumb polydactyly may be sporadic, usually transmitted as an autosomal dominant trait with variable expressivity. A similar clinical picture can be seen in the big toe with bifurcation of the terminal phalanx and duplication of the nail. Early treatment is important to maximize functional restoration and aesthetical results.

Worn down and shiny nails

Patients with atopic dermatitis or chronic erythroderma may be 'chronic scratchers and rubbers'. The surface of the nail plate becomes glossy and shiny and the free edge is worn away (Figures 2.39, 2.40). Thus *usure*

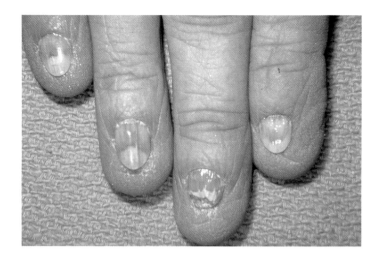

Figure 2.35

Micronychia – 'small nail field' defect in hidrotic ectodermal dysplasia. (Courtesy of L. Norton.)

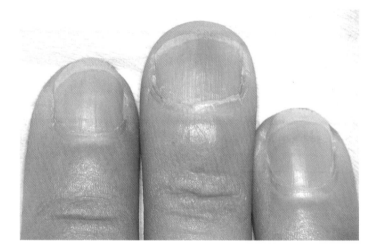

Figure 2.36

Macronychia – middle finger.

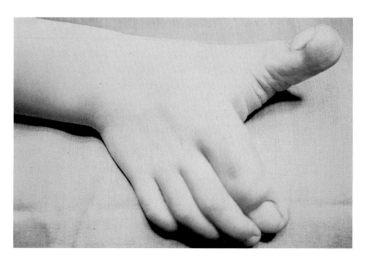

Figure 2.37

Macronychia with macrodactyly – Proteus syndrome.

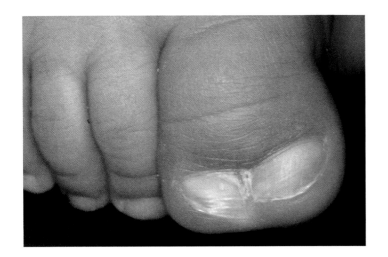

Figure 2.38

Bifid toe.

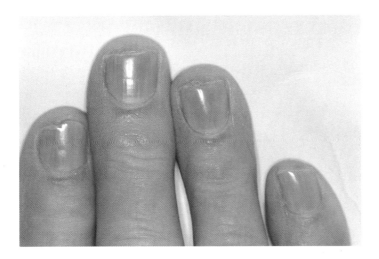

Figure 2.39

Worn down shiny nails (*usure des ongles*), due to chronic rubbing and scratching.

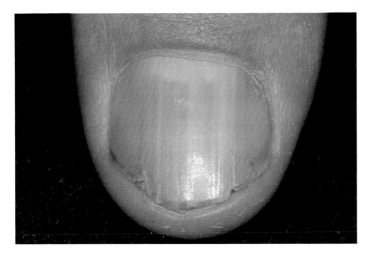

Figure 2.40

Darier's disease – worn down tips due to intrinsic keratinization defect; note associated white lines.

> **Shiny nails of the hands usually implies severe scratching or rubbing of skin**

des ongles may also occur in many different manual occupations. It has recently been described as a particular hazard of individuals handling heavy plastic bags.

Worn down nails: occupational causes

Smooth	Atopic eczema
Shiny nails	Pruritic lymphoma
	Chronic pruritus
Distal	Trauma
fraying	Darier's disease
	Old age
	Nail scratchers

Anonychia and onychatrophy

It is quite impossible to differentiate completely these two signs in the light of current knowledge. In principle the term 'anonychia' (total or partial) is probably best reserved for conditions in which the nail has failed to develop; 'onychatrophy' should be used to describe processes in which the nail has initially formed satisfactorily and then shown total or partial regression. Table 2.7 lists the causes of anonychia and onychatrophy.

In aplastic anonychia, a rare congenital disorder occasionally associated with other defects such as ectrodactyly, the nail never forms. Loose horny masses are produced by the metaplastic, squamous epithelium of the matrix and the nail bed in anonychia keratodes. Hypoplasia of the nail plates is a hallmark of the nail–patella syndrome; in the

Table 2.7   Causes of anonychia and onychatrophy

Permanent hypo- or anonychia (Figures 2.41–2.43)
+/– ectrodactyly
+/– dental malformations
Nail–patella syndrome (Figure 2.44)
Congenital onychodysplasia of index
    finger
Coffin–Siris syndrome with many congenital
    defects
DOOR syndrome (deafness, onycho-
    osteodystrophy, mental retardation)

Onychatrophy (Figures 2.45–2.53)
With pterygium (Figure 2.50)
    Lichen planus (Figure 2.50)
    Acrosclerosis (Figure 2.47)
    Onychotillomania (Figures 2.52, 2.53)
    Lesch–Nyhan syndrome
    Chronic graft versus host disease
    Stevens–Johnson and Lyell syndrome
    Cicatricial pemphigoid

Without pterygium
    Severe paronychia with nail dystrophy
    Stevens–Johnson or Lyell syndrome
    Epidermolysis bullosa (Figure 2.48)
    Amyloidosis
    Etretinate nail dystrophy (Figure 2.46)
    Idiopathic atrophy of childhood
    Severe psoriatic nail dystrophy (Figure 2.49)

---

least affected cases only the ulnar half of each thumb nail is missing.

Onychatrophy presents as a reduction in size and thickness of the nail plate, often accompanied by fragmentation and splitting, for example in lichen planus. It may progressively worsen, scar tissue eventually replacing the atrophic nail plate.

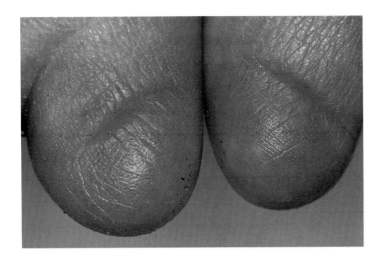

Figure 2.41

Congenital absence of nails.

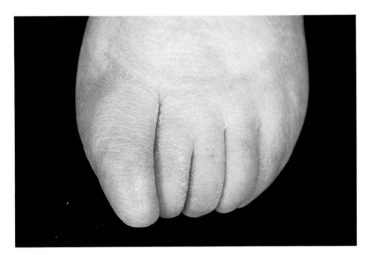

Figure 2.42

Congenital absence of nails in the DOOR syndrome. (Courtesy of Professor Nevin, Belfast.)

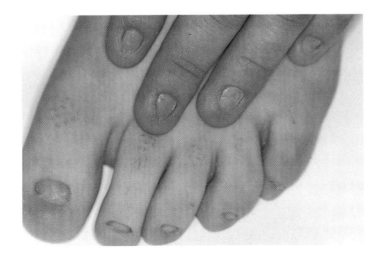

Figure 2.43

Micronychia in congenital ectodermal dysplasia.

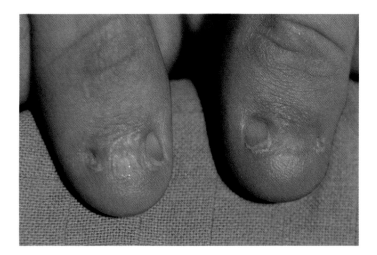

Figure 2.44

Partial anonychia in the nail–patella syndrome.

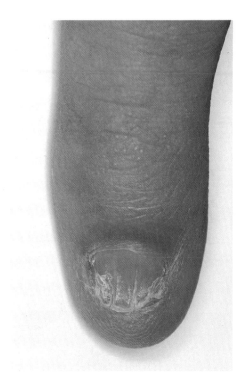

Figure 2.45

Onychatrophy – ectodermal dysplasia.

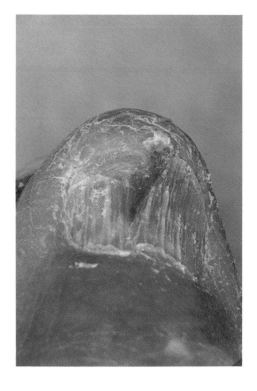

Figure 2.46

Onychatrophy due to oral Etretinate therapy. (Courtesy of B. Kalis, Reims)

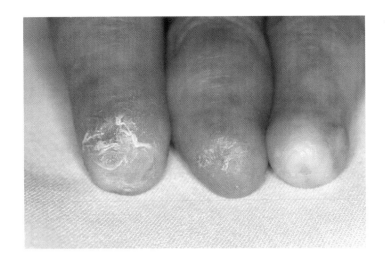

Figure 2.47

Onychatrophy – acrosclerosis.

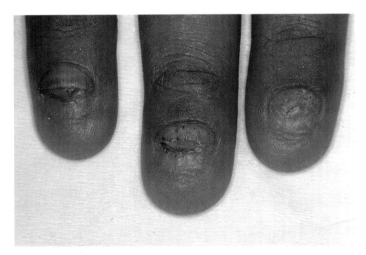

Figure 2.48

Onychatrophy – epidermolysis bullosa.

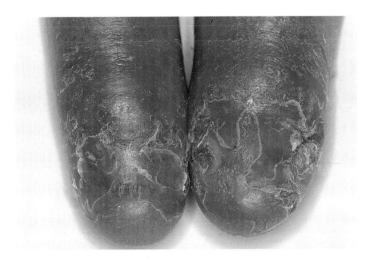

Figure 2.49

Onychatrophy – pustular psoriasis.

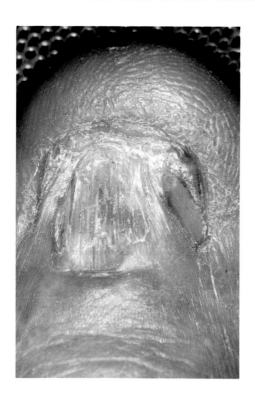

Figure 2.50
Onychatrophy – lichen planus.

Further reading

Clubbing

Dickinson CJ, Martin JF (1987) Megakaryocytes and platelet clumps as the cause of finger clubbing, *Lancet* ii: 1434–1435.

Fischer DS, Singer DH, Feldman SM (1964) Clubbing, a review, with emphasis on hereditary acropachy, *Medicine* 43: 459–479.

Koilonychia

Hogan GR, Jones B (1970) The relationship between koilonychia and iron deficiency in infants, *J Pediatr* 77: 1054–1057.

Stone OJ (1985) Clubbing and koilonychia, *Dermatol Clin* 3: 485–490.

Transverse overcurvature

Cornelius CE, Shelley WB (1968) Pincer nail syndrome, *Arch Surg* 96: 321–322.

Cohen P, Milewicz DM (1993) Dolichonychia in a patient with the Marfan syndrome, *J Dermatol* 20: 779–782.

Haneke E (1992) Etiopathogénie et traitement de l'hypercourbure transversale de l'ongle du gros orteil, *J Méd Esth Chir Dermatol* 19: 123–127.

Brachyonychia

Rubinstein JH (1969) The broad thumbs syndrome progress report 1968, *Birth Defects: Original Article Series* V(2): 25–41.

Micro- and macronychia

Kikuchi I (1985) Congenital polyonychias: reduction versus duplication digit malformations, *Int J Dermatol* 24: 211–215.

Telfer NR, Barth JH, Dawber RPR (1988) Congenital and hereditary nail dystrophies: an embryological approach to classification, *Clin Exp Dermatol* 13: 160–163.

Anonychia and nail atrophy

Zaias N (1970) The nail in lichen planus, *Arch Dermatol* 101: 264–271.

Polydactyly

Tosti A, Paoluzzi P, Baran R (1992) Doubled nail of the thumb: a rare form of polydactyly, *Dermatology* 184: 216–218.

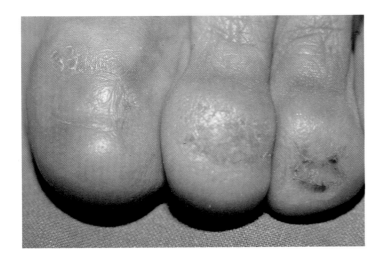

Figure 2.51

Onychatrophy – lichen planus with total nail loss.

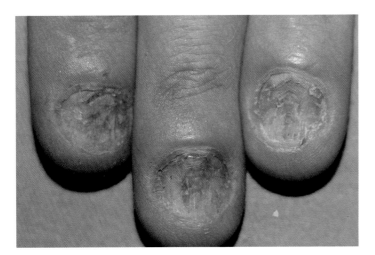

Figure 2.52

Onychatrophy – severe nail biting.

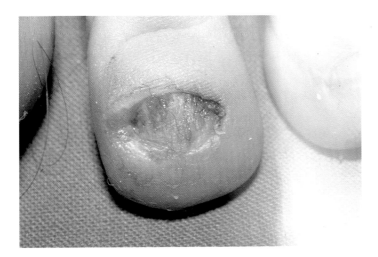

Figure 2.53

Onychatrophy – onychotillomania.

3 Modifications of nail surface

Longitudinal lines

Longitudinal lines, or striations, may appear as indented grooves or projecting ridges (Figures 3.1–3.8).

Longitudinal grooves

Longitudinal grooves represent long-lasting abnormalities and can develop under the following conditions:

A single longitudinal nail fissure is most likely due to minor trauma

1 Physiological, as shallow and delicate furrows, usually parallel, and separated by low, projecting ridges. They become more prominent with age and in certain pathological states, such as lichen planus (Figure 3.4), rheumatoid arthritis, peripheral vascular (arterial) insufficiency,

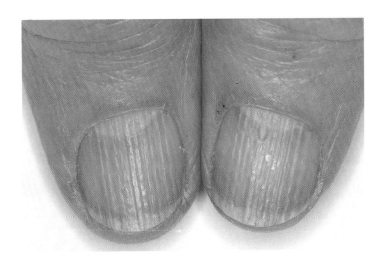

Figure 3.1

Longitudinal lines – associated with old age.

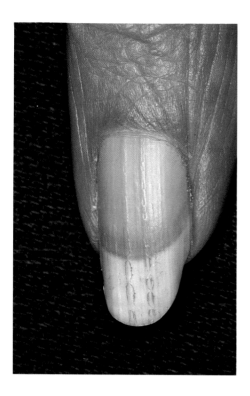

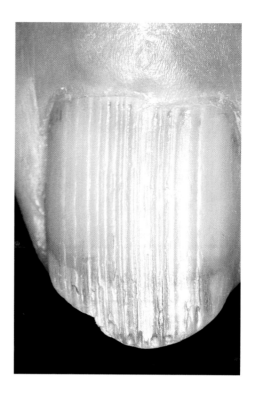

Figure 3.2

Longitudinal lines – old age 'sausage link' appearance.

Figure 3.3

Longitudinal lines – prominent old age changes, which may occur earlier with chronic arterial impairment.

Darier's disease and other genetic abnormalities.

2   Onychorrhexis consists of a series of narrow, longitudinal, parallel superficial furrows with the appearance of having been scratched by an awl. Sometimes dust becomes ingrained into the nail surface. Splitting of the free edge is common.

3   Tumours, such as myxoid cysts and warts, in the proximal nail fold area may exert pressure on the nail matrix and produce a wide, deep, longitudinal groove or canal, which disappears if the cause is removed (Figure 3.8).

4   Median nail dystrophy (Figure 3.7). This uncommon condition consists of a longitudinal defect of the thumb nails in the mid-line or just off centre, starting at the cuticle and growing out of the free edge. It may be associated with an enlarged lunula. In early descriptions, the base of the 2 to 5 mm wide groove with steep edges showed numerous transverse defects. More recent reports have shown longitudinal fissures as *dystrophia longi-*

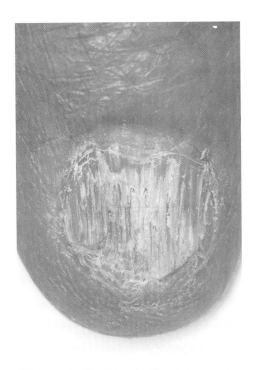

Figure 3.4

Longitudinal dystrophy in lichen planus.

tudinalis fissuriformis. In some cases median longitudinal ridges have been observed, occasionally combined with fissures and/or a groove, developed from the distal edge of the nail plate to the matrix. Often a few short feathery cracks, chevron-shaped, extend laterally from the split – the 'inverted fir tree' appearance. The so-called naevus striatus symmetricus of the thumbs corresponds to this form. Median nail dystrophy is usually symmetrical and most often affects the thumbs. Sometimes other fingers are involved, the toes less commonly (usually the big toe). After several months or years, the nail returns to normal but recurrences are not rare. Familial cases have been recorded. The aetiology is unknown, although it has been suggested that it is due to self-inflicted trauma resulting from a tic or habit. Treatment of recalcitrant cases may be identical to post-traumatic nail splitting.

5   A central longitudinal depression is found in 'washboard nail plates' caused

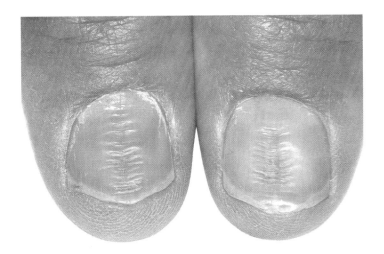

Figure 3.5

Central longitudinal grooved dystrophy – self-induced by trauma to the matrix.

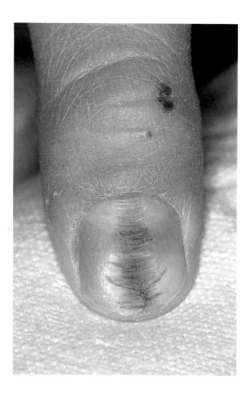

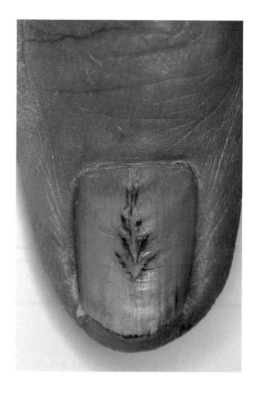

Figure 3.6

Self-induced deep groove plus transverse lines – self-induced matrix trauma.

Figure 3.7

Heller's median canaliform dystrophy.

by chronic, mechanical injury (Figures 3.5–3.6). Unlike median nail dystrophy (Heller's dystrophy), the cuticle is pushed back and there is accompanying inflammation and/or thickening of the proximal nail fold. Splits due to trauma, or those occurring in the nail–patella syndrome and in pterygium, are usually obvious. Longitudinal splits may also result from Raynaud's disease, lichen striatus and trachyonychia.

Nail wrapping (Chapter 9) may lessen the disability produced by the fissure; the proximal nail fold must be protected from repeated minor trauma.

Longitudinal ridges

Small rectilinear projections extend from the proximal nail fold as far as the free edge of the nail; or they may stop short. They may be interrupted at regular intervals, giving rise to a beaded appearance. Sometimes a wide, longitudinal median ridge has the appearance, in cross-section, of a circumflex accent.

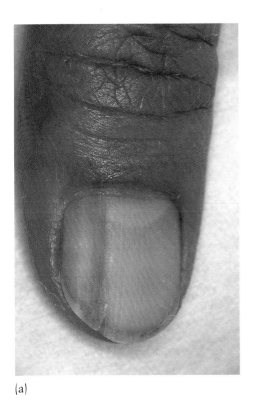

(a)

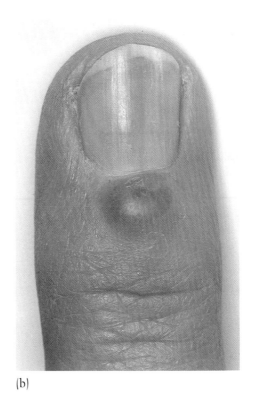

(b)

Figure 3.8

Longitudinal nail groove due to (a) glomus tumour, (b) myxoid cyst.

It is inherited and affects mainly the thumb and index fingers of both hands.

Table 3.1 shows the principal causes of longitudinal lines and grooves.

Herringbone nails

This pattern of nail ridging, with oblique lines pointing centrally to meet in the midline, has been reported as an uncommon phenomenon occurring in childhood (Figure 3.9). It characteristically disappears as the child grows. Less obvious, similar lines may be seen associated with the pointed matrix of the nail–patella syndrome.

Transverse lines

Transverse, band-like depressions extending from one lateral edge of the nail to the other, and affecting all nails at corresponding

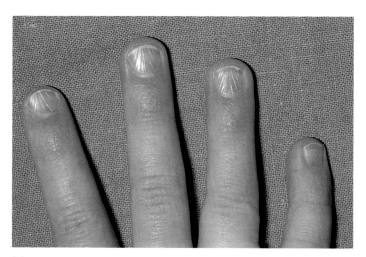

(a)

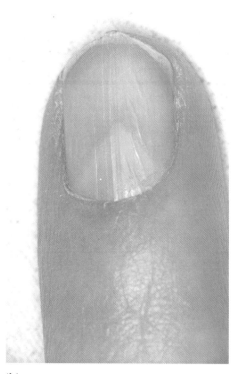

(b)

Figure 3.9

(a) Herringbone nail appearance with oblique lines meeting in the midline – a temporary change of early childhood; (b) nail–patella syndrome – more subtle, but similar lines to (a); associated with pointed lunula. (Figure 3.9 (a) from Parry EJ, Morley WN, Dawber RPR (1995), Herringbone nails: an uncommon variant of nail growth in childhood? *Br J Dermatol* **132**: 1021–1022.)

Table 3.1   Causes of longitudinal lines

Coloured lines

White	*See* leukonychia (pages 140–146)
Black	*See* melanonychia (pages 147–153)
Red	Darier's disease (*see* Figure 2.40)
	Vascular tumours
	Glomus (Figure 3.8)
	Cirsoid

Linear ridges

Single	Familial
	Median canaliform dystrophy (Figure 3.7)
	Trauma (isolated or repeated)
	Tumours
Multiple	Normal – increase with age after early adulthood (Figures 3.2, 3.3)
	With all causes of thin nail plates
	Lichen planus (Figure 3.4)
	Rheumatoid arthritis
	Graft-versus-host disease
	Psoriasis
	Darier's disease
	Poor circulation
	Collagen vascular diseases
	Radiation
	Frostbite
	Alopecia areata
	Nail–patella syndrome

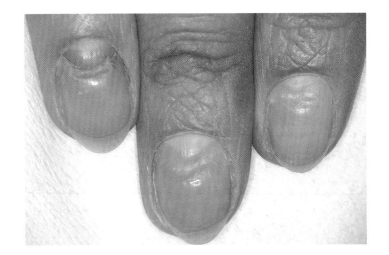

Figure 3.10

Beau's lines.

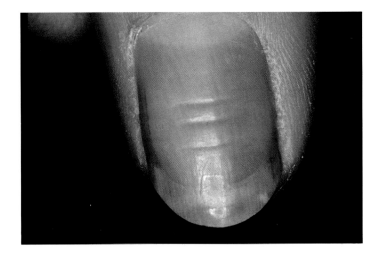

Figure 3.11

Transverse lines due to chemotherapy cycles. (Courtesy of L. Requena.)

levels, are called Beau's lines (Figures 3.10–3.13). They may be noted after any severe, sudden acute, particularly febrile illness. In milder cases the nails of the thumb and the big toe are the most reliable markers, as the former would supply information for the previous 6 to 9 months and the latter would show evidence of disease for up to 2 years (relating to the different rates of linear nail growth).

> **Beau's lines on all 20 nails is usually the result of systemic disease**

The width of the transverse groove relates to the duration of the disease which has affected the matrix. The distal limit of the furrow, if abrupt, indicates a sudden attack of disease, if sloping, a more protracted

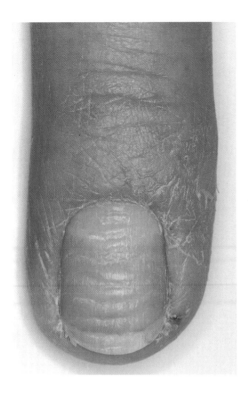

Figure 3.12

Beau's lines – psoriasis.

onset. In fact the proximal limit of the depression may be abrupt and both limits may well be sloped.

If the duration of the disease can completely inhibit the activity of the matrix for 1 to 2 weeks or longer, the transverse depression will result in total division of the nail plate, a defect known as 'onychomadesis' (Figures 3.14, 3.15). As the nail adheres firmly to the nail bed the onychomadesis remains latent for several weeks before leading to temporary shedding.

Transverse furrows may be due to measles in childhood, zinc deficiency (often multiple), Stevens–Johnson and Lyell's syndromes, cytotoxic drugs and many other non-specific events. Beau's lines can also be physiological, e.g. marks appearing with each menstrual cycle, particularly in dysmenorrhoea. They have also been noted in 4- to 5-week-old babies without any obvious cause.

When only a few digits are involved this may indicate trauma, carpal tunnel syndrome, chronic paronychia or chronic eczema. If they follow a chronic condition, the lines are often numerous and curvilinear.

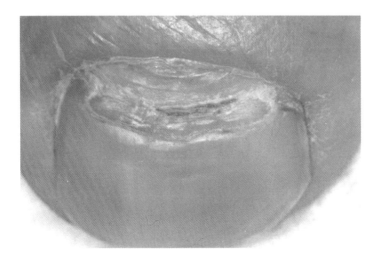

Figure 3.13

Long Beau's line (depression) due to more prolonged arrest of growth. (Courtesy of J.P. Ortonne, Nice)

When a series of transverse grooves parallels the proximal nail fold the cause is likely to be repeated trauma from over-zealous manicuring. 'Rhythmic' parallel transverse grooves may be an isolated sign of psoriasis, equivalent to patterned pitting.

The nervous habit of pushing back the cuticle usually affects the thumbs which are damaged by either the thumb nail of the opposite hand or the index finger nail of the corresponding hand: symmetrical involvement of the thumbs is the rule and damage is most commonly effected by the thumb nail of the other hand (Figures 3.5, 3.6). Occasionally only one thumb is affected; rarely, other digits may be involved, the thumb reversing roles and creating the damage. This produces:

1 Swelling, redness and scaling of the proximal nail fold from the mechanical injury
2 Multiple horizontal grooves that do not extend to the lateral margin of the nail; often filled with debris, they are interspersed between the ridges

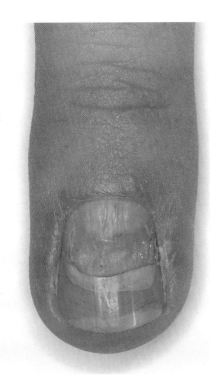

Figure 3.14

Onychomadesis – in this case due to bleomycin therapy for warts on the proximal nail fold.

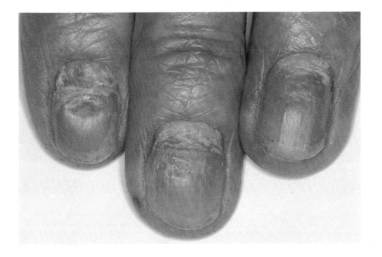

Figure 3.15

Beau's lines/onychomadesis – due to psoriasis.

Table 3.2   Causes of transverse grooves

Common
  High fever
  Postnatal
  Menstrual cycle (multiple), dysmenorrhoea
  Measles
  Trauma
  Chronic paronychia
  Local inflammation
  Chronic eczema

Uncommon
  Kawasaki syndrome
  Stevens–Johnson syndrome
  Cytotoxic drugs
  Acrodermatitis enteropathica and zinc
    deficiency
  Hypoparathyroidism
  Syphilis

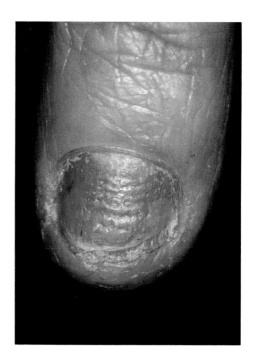

3   A large central longitudinal or slightly lateral depression along the nail mimicking median canaliform dystrophy, with an enlarged lunula.

Table 3.2 lists causes of transverse groove formation.

Figure 3.16

Multiple nail pits – arranged in transverse lines.

Pitting and rippling

> **Occasional nail pits are due to minor trauma. Profuse pitting is most often due to psoriasis**

Pitting and rippling are also known as pits, onychia punctata, erosions and Rosenau's depressions. Pits develop as a result of defective nail formation in punctate areas located in the proximal portion of the nail matrix. The surface of the nail plate is studded with small punctate depressions which vary in number, size, depth and shape. The depth and width of the pits relates to the extent of the matrix involved; their length is determined by the duration of the matrix damage. They may be randomly distributed or uniformly arranged in series along one or several longitudinal lines; they are sometimes arranged in a criss-cross pattern and may resemble the external surface of a thimble.

It has been shown that regular pitting may convert to rippling or ridging and these

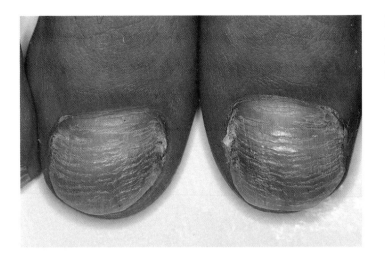

Figure 3.17

Multiple nail pits – similar to Figure 3.16, but more lined in appearance.

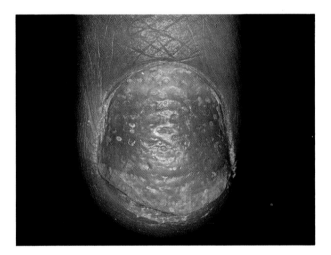

Figure 3.18

Multiple nail pits – due to psoriasis.

two conditions appear, at times, to be variants of uniform pitting (Figures 3.16, 3.17). Nails showing diffuse pitting grow faster than the apparently normal nails in psoriasis. Occasional pits occur on normal nails. Deep pits can be attributed to psoriasis (Figure 3.18). In alopecia areata (Figure 3.19) shallow pits are usually seen and they are quite often very numerous, leading to trachyonychia (rough nail) and twenty nail dystrophy; however, curiously, one nail often remains unaffected for a long time. Pits may also occur in eczema or occupational trauma. In some cases a genetic basis is thought likely. In secondary syphilis and pityriasis rosea pitting occurs rarely. We have observed one case of the latter, with the pits distributed on all the finger nails at corresponding levels, analogous to Beau's lines.

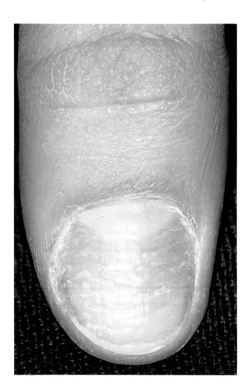

Figure 3.19

Multiple nail pits – 'rippled' effect in alopecia areata.

Table 3.3 lists the commonest causes of nail pitting.

Trachyonychia (rough nails)

The term twenty nail dystrophy or trachyonychia, describes a spectrum of nail plate surface abnormalities that result in nail roughness. Patients with trachyonychia can be divided into two main groups:

Table 3.3   Causes of pitting

Common
  Psoriasis (Figures 3.16–3.18, 3.20)
  Alopecia areata (Figure 3.19)
  Eczema
  Occupational trauma
  Parakeratosis pustulosa

Uncommon
  Normal
  Pityriasis rosea
  Secondary syphilis
  Sarcoidosis
  Reiter's syndrome
  Lichen planus

1   Trachyonychia and a past history or clinical evidence of alopecia areata.
2   Isolated nail involvement (idiopathic trachyonychia). Twenty nail dystrophy usually occurs sporadically but a few familial and hereditary cases have been reported. It has occasionally been described in association with ichthyosis vulgaris and atopic dermatitis, diffuse neurodermatitis, vitiligo, dark red lunulae and knuckle pads, selective IgA deficiency, autoimmune thrombocytopenic purpura and haemolytic anaemia.

Trachyonychia occurs in approximately 12% of children and 3.3% of adults with alopecia areata. It is more frequent in males than in females and in patients with alope-

> **Idiopathic trachyonychia of childhood is a benign condition that usually returns entirely to normal**

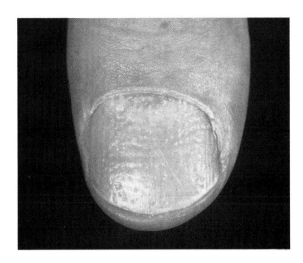

Figure 3.20

Diffuse pitting of the whole nail in psoriasis.

Table 3.4 **Causes and associations of trachyonychia**

Common
  Idiopathic (twenty nail dystrophy)
  Alopecia areata (Figures 3.21, 3.22)
  Lichen planus (Figures 3.23, 3.24)
  Eczematous histology
  Chemicals

Less common
  Ichthyosis vulgaris
  Ectodermal dysplasias
  Selective IgA deficiency
  Knuckle pads and dark lunulae
  Amyloidosis (systemic)

cia totalis or universalis as compared with patients with patchy hair loss. The onset of trachyonychia may precede or follow the onset of alopecia areata, even by years. It is most usual for hair loss and nail changes to develop concurrently.

The frequency of idiopathic trachyonychia is unknown, although it is certainly rare, more commonly but not exclusively seen in children. Idiopathic trachyonychia may be a clinical manifestation of several nail diseases including lichen planus, psoriasis, eczema and

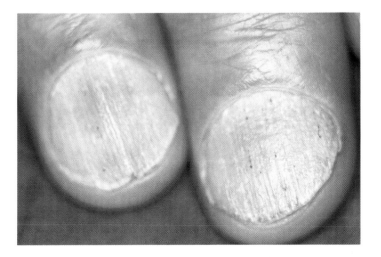

Figure 3.21

Trachyonychia (rough nails) – due to alopecia areata.

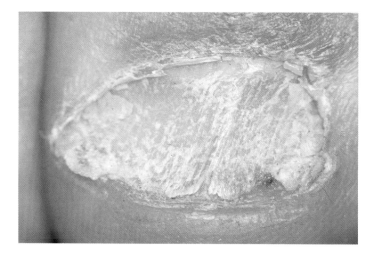

Figure 3.22
Trachyonychia – idiopathic.

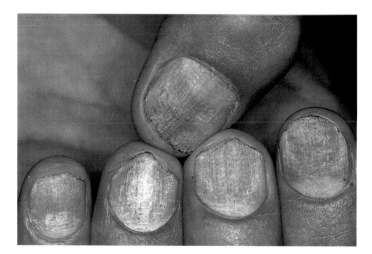

Figure 3.23
Trachyonychia – lichen planus.

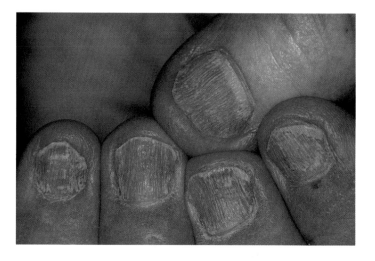

Figure 3.24
Trachyonychia – twenty nail dystrophy of lichen planus.

pemphigus vulgaris. It may also represent a clinical variety of alopecia areata limited to the nails. Two clinical varieties of trachyonychia have been described: opaque trachyonychia and shiny trachyonychia. Both these varieties may occur in association with alopecia areata or may be idiopathic. Opaque trachyonychia is more common than the shiny type.

In opaque trachyonychia the nail plate surface shows severe longitudinal ridging and is covered by multiple adherent small scales. The nail is thin, opaque, lustreless and gives the impression of having been sandpapered in a longitudinal direction (vertically striated sandpapered nails). The cuticle of the affected nails is ragged and some degree of koilonychia is often present. In shiny trachyonychia, the nail plate surface abnormalities are less severe. Nail plate roughness is mild and caused by a myriad of minuscule punctate depressions, which give the nail plate surface a shiny appearance. In some patients a proportion of the nails have the sandpapered appearance while others have the shiny appearance. Trachyonychia is symptomless and patients only complain of brittleness and cosmetic discomfort.

Although trachyonychia is better known as twenty nail dystrophy, the nail changes do not necessarily involve all 20 nails in every patient. It is a nail symptom which may be caused by several inflammatory diseases that disturb nail matrix keratinization. There are no clinical criteria that enable one to distinguish spongiotic trachyonychia, the most common type, from trachyonychia due to other inflammatory skin diseases, i.e. lichen planus, psoriasis, eczema, or pemphigus vulgaris. Trachyonychia is a benign condition that never produces nail scarring. This is true not only for trachyonychia associated with spongiotic changes, but also for trachyonychia due to lichen planus or other dermatological diseases. Spongiotic trachyonychia regresses spontaneously in a few years in most patients.

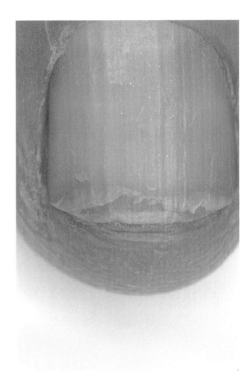

Figure 3.25

Onychoschizia (lamellar splitting or layering).

Table 3.4 lists the known causes and associations of trachyonychia.

Onychoschizia (lamellar splitting)

'Layering' in the distal portion of the finger nail is usually due to frequent wetting

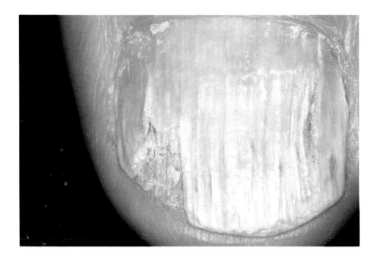

Figure 3.26
Onychoschizia and onychorrhexis due to lichen planus.

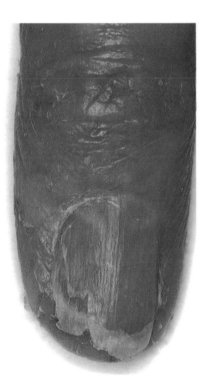

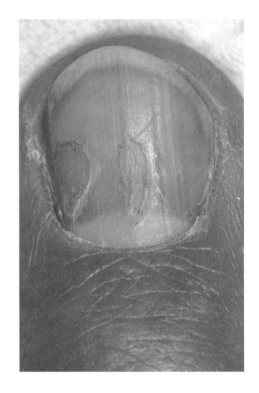

Figure 3.27
Onychoschizia due to oral retinoid therapy.

Figure 3.28
More proximal onychoschizia due to oral retinoids.

Table 3.5   Causes of lamellar splitting

Proximal
    Psoriasis
    Lichen planus (Figure 3.26)
    Retinoid therapy (Figure 3.27)

Distal
    Chemical injury
    Old age
    Repeated nailwetting
    Chondrodysplasia punctata – X-linked
    Polycythaemia vera

In this condition, the distal portion of the nail splits horizontally. The nail is formed in layers somewhat analogous to plywood and the formation of scales in the epidermis (Figure 3.25). Various exogenous factors may contribute to the defect. It is common in housewives and others whose nails are repeatedly soaked in water, leading to frequent hydration and dehydration. Splitting into layers has been reported in X-linked dominant chondrodysplasia punctata and in polycythaemia vera. The onychoschizia may be seen in the proximal portion of the nail in lichen planus (Figure 3.26) and also as a result of oral retinoid therapy (Figures 3.27, 3.28).

Table 3.5 lists the known causes of onychoschizia.

Further reading

Herringbone nails

Parry EJ, Morley WN, Dawber RPR (1995) Herringbone nails: an uncommon variant of nail growth in childhood? *Br J Dermatol* **132**: 1021–1022.

Trachyonychia

Baran R, Dawber RPR (1987) Twenty nail dystrophy of childhood: a misnamed syndrome, *Cutis* **39**: 481–482.
Tosti A, Fanti PA, Morelli R, Bardazzi F (1991) Trachyonychia associated with alopecia areata: a clinical and pathological study, *J Am Acad Dermatol* **25**: 266–270.
Tosti A, Bardazzi F, Piraccini BM, Fanti PA (1994) Trachyonychia (twenty nail dystrophy): clinical and pathological study of 23 patients, *Br J Dermatol* **131**: 866–872.

Onychoschizia

Shelley WB, Shelley ED (1984) Onychoschizia: scanning electron microscopy, *J Am Acad Dermatol* **10**: 623-627.

4 Nail plate and soft tissue abnormalities

Onycholysis

Onycholysis refers to the detachment of the nail from its bed at its distal and/or lateral attachments (Figure 4.1).

The pattern of separation of the plate from the nail bed takes many forms. Sometimes it resembles closely the damage from a splinter under the nail, the detachment extending proximally along a convex line, giving the appearance of a half-moon. When the process reaches the matrix, onycholysis becomes complete. Involvement of the lateral edge of the nail plate alone is less common. In certain cases, the free edge rises up like a hood, or coils upon itself like a roll of paper. Onycholysis creates a subungual space that gathers dirt and keratinous debris; the greyish-white colour is due to the presence of air under the nail but the colour may vary from yellow to brown, depending on the aetiology. This area is sometimes malodorous.

In psoriasis (Figures 4.2–4.4) there is usually a yellowish-brown margin visible between the pink, normal nail and the white, separated area. In the 'oil spot' or 'salmon-patch' variety, the nail plate–nail bed separation may start in the middle of the nail; this

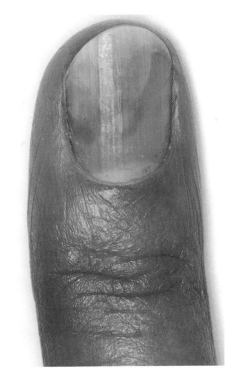

Figure 4.1

Onycholysis.

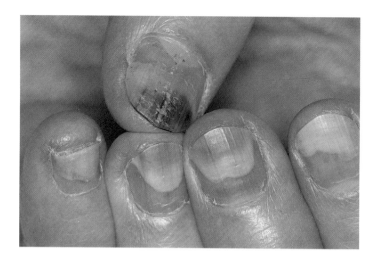

Figure 4.2

Onycholysis – with *Pseudomonas pyocyanea* discoloration.

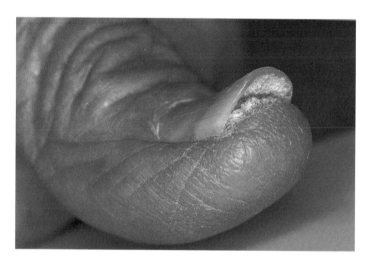

Figure 4.3

Onycholysis – showing the separation of the nail plate and nail bed.

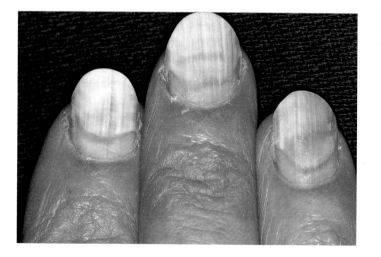

Figure 4.4

Onycholysis due to psoriasis.

is sometimes surrounded by a yellow margin, especially in psoriasis. The accumulation of large amounts of serum-like exudate containing glycoprotein, in and under the affected nails, explains the colour change in this kind of onycholysis. Glycoprotein deposition is commonly found in inflammatory and eczematous diseases affecting the nail bed. Oil patches have been reported in systemic lupus erythematosus; they may be extensive in lectitis purulenta et granulomatosa.

Onycholysis is usually symptomless and it is mainly the appearance of the nail which brings the patient to the doctor; occasionally there is slight pain associated with inflammation in the early stages. The extent of onycholysis increases progressively and can be estimated by measuring the distance separating the distal edge of the lunula from the proximal limit detachment. Transillumination of the terminal phalanx gives a good view of the affected area.

Finger nail onycholysis as an isolated sign on a few nails in adult women is often perpetuated by 'introspective' overzealous manicuring

The onset may be sudden, as in photo-onycholysis (Figure 4.5) where there may be a triad of photosensitization, onycholysis and dyschromia, and when it is due to contact with chemical irritants such as hydrofluoric acid. Sculptured onycholysis is a self-induced nail abnormality produced by cleaning the underside of the nail plate with a sharp instrument; this results in an opaque, distal portion of the nail with a gently curved, proximal, 'lytic' border.

Onycholysis of the toe demonstrates some differences from the condition on the fingers: the major distinctions are due to:

- The lack of occupational factors
- The reduced use of cosmetics on the feet

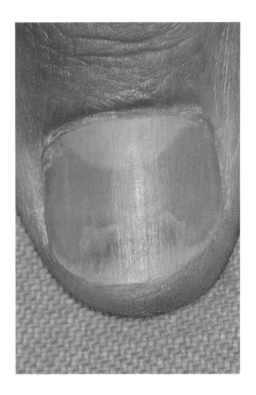

Figure 4.5

Photo-onycholysis.

- The protection afforded by footwear which reduces the risk of photo-onycholysis.

The two main causes of onycholysis of the toe nail, especially the great toe nail, are onychomycosis and traumatic onycholysis. Onycholysis of the great toe nail is often seen when the second toe overrides it. Other causes are onychogryphosis and, in children, congenital malalignment of the hallux nails. In both cases, the nail is thickened, discoloured, brittle and deviates from the normal axis. A blunt probe can be inserted under the nail plate up to the matrix without

Table 4.1   Some causes of onycholysis

Idiopathic
  Leuko-onycholysis paradentotica (Schuppli syndrome)
  Of women (probably cosmetic)

Systemic
  Circulatory (e.g. lupus erythematosus)
  Yellow nail syndrome
  Endocrine (e.g. hypothyroidism, thyrotoxicosis)
  Pregnancy
  Syphilis
  Iron deficiency anaemia
  Carcinoma of the lung
  Pellagra

Congenital and/or hereditary
  Partial hereditary onycholysis
  Pachyonychia congenita

Cutaneous diseases
  Psoriasis, Reiter's disease, vesicular or bullous disease, lichen planus, alopecia areata, multicentric
    reticulohistiocytosis
  Atopic dermatitis, contact dermatitis (accidental or occupational), mycosis fungoides, actinic
    reticuloid
  Hyperhidrosis – tumours of the nail bed
  Drugs: bleomycin, doxorubicin, 5-fluorouracil, retinoids, captopril
  Drug-induced photo-onycholysis: trypaflavine, chlorpromazine, chloramphenicol, cephaloridine,
    cloxacillin (exceptional), tetracyclines: especially demethylchlortetracycline and doxycycline, also
    minocycline, photochemotherapy with psoralens (sunlight or PUVA), thiazide, diuretics,
    flumequine, quinine

Local causes
  Traumatic (accidental, occupational, self-inflicted (Figure 4.6) or mixed) as with clawing, pinching
    or stabbing
  Foreign bodies
  Infectious
    Fungal
    Bacterial
    Viral (e.g. warts, herpes simplex, herpes zoster)
  Chemical (accidental or occupational)
  Prolonged immersion in (hot) water with alkalis and/or detergents, sodium hypochlorite, etc.
  Paint removers
  Sugar solution
  Gasoline and similar solvents
  Cosmetics (formaldehyde, false nails, depilatory products, nail polish removers). Nickel derived
    from metal pellets in nail varnish
  Physical
  Thermal injury (accidental or occupational)
  Microwaves

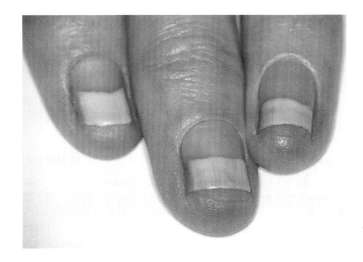

Figure 4.6

Self-induced onycholysis.

causing pain. The nail bed epithelium is irreversibly transformed into epidermis, thus prohibiting reattachment of the nail.

Primary *Candida* onycholysis is almost exclusively confined to the finger nails. In distal subungual onychomycosis of the toe nails, the horny thickening raises the free edge of the nail with disruption of the normal nail plate–nail bed attachment; this gives rise to secondary onycholysis. Some authors have questioned whether big toe nail onychomycosis is ever truly primary. Its presence should always lead to a search for abnormalities of the foot such as hyperkeratosis of the metatarsal heads, thickening of the ball of the foot or pressure on the big toe by an overriding second toe.

Table 4.1 lists many potential causes of onycholysis. The commonest types presenting to dermatologists are due to psoriasis, onychomycosis and the cosmetic 'sculptured' varieties of adult women.

Onychomadesis and shedding

Nails may be shed by the progression of any severe type of onycholysis causing the nail plate to separate more proximally. Onychomadesis is the spontaneous separation of the nail plate from the matrix area; this is associated with some arrest of nail growth (*see* the section on transverse lines, Chapter 3). At first, a split appears under the proximal portion of the nail followed by the disappearance of the juxtamatricial portion of the surface of the nail. A surface defect is thus formed, which does not usually involve the deeper layers. It is due to a 'limited' lesion of the proximal part of the matrix.

In latent onychomadesis the nail plate shows a transverse split because of transient, complete inhibition of nail growth for a minimum of 1 to 2 weeks. It may be characterized by a Beau's line which has reached its maximum dimensions, although the nail continues growing for some time because there is no disruption in its attachment to the underlying tissues. Growth ceases when it is shed after losing this connection. In some very severe, general acute diseases, such as Lyell's syndrome, the proximal edge of all the nail plates may be elevated. Growth proceeds because of the continued movement of the nail bed to which the nails remain attached.

The terms onychoptosis defluvium or alopecia unguium are sometimes used to describe traumatic nail loss. Onychomadesis usually results from serious generalized diseases, bullous dermatoses, drug reactions, intensive X-ray therapy, acute paronychia or severe psychological stress; or it may be idiopathic. Nail shedding may be an inherited disorder (as a dominant trait); the shedding may be periodic, and rarely associated with the dental condition amelogenesis imperfecta. Longitudinal fissures, recurrent onychomadesis and onychogryphosis can be associated with mild degrees of keratosis punctata. Minor traumatic episodes (as in sportsman's toe) may cause onychomadesis of the toe nails.

Total nail loss with scarring may be due to permanent damage of the matrix following trauma, or the late stages of acquired onychatrophy following lichen planus, bullous diseases or chronic peripheral vascular insufficiency. In texts on congenital anomalies, this defect is sometimes referred to as aplastic anonychia, which does not always produce scarring. Temporary, total nail loss may also result from severe progressive onycholysis.

Table 4.2 lists many of the recognized causes of nail shedding.

Table 4.2   Causes and associations of nail shedding

Local inflammation, e.g. acute paronychia
  (Figures 4.7–4.12)
Kawasaki syndrome
Fever/systemic upsets
Syphilis
Bullous dermatoses, e.g. pemphigus
Stevens–Johnson syndrome
Lyell's syndrome (Figures 4.7–4.9)
Drugs
  Cytotoxics
  Antibiotics
  Retinoids
Keratosis punctata
Local trauma
X-irradiation
Acrodermatitis enteropathica
Hypoparathyroidism with amelogenesis
  imperfecta
Yellow nail syndrome

Hypertrophy and subungual hyperkeratosis

Ideally, the term 'hypertrophy of the nail plate' should be restricted to those conditions causing nail enlargement and thickening by their effects on the nail matrix (excluding nail bed and hyponychium). 'Subungual hyperkeratosis' should relate to those entities leading to thickening beneath the preformed nail plate, that is, thickening of the nail bed or hyponychium (Figure 4.13). In practice, this differentiation is difficult to define and mixed cases are commonly seen, for example in psoriasis (Figures 4.14, 4.15).

The normal thickness of finger nails is approximately 0.5 mm; this is consistently increased in manual workers and in many disease states such as congenital ichthyoses, Darier's disease, psoriasis and repeated trauma. The latter particularly relates to toe nails where microtrauma and footwear are constantly affecting the nails.

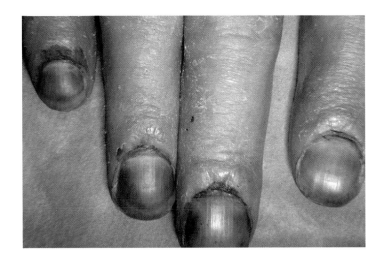

Figure 4.7

Lyell's syndrome – early proximal changes.

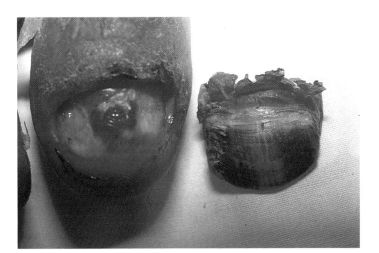

Figure 4.8

Lyell's syndrome – nail shedding. (Courtesy of S. Goettmann.)

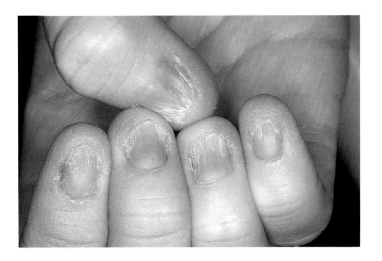

Figure 4.9

Lyell's syndrome – nails shed and permanent scarring. (Courtesy of S. Goettmann.)

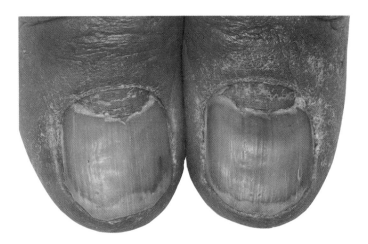

Figure 4.10

Onychomadesis due to psoriasis.

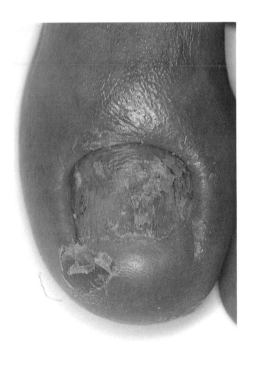

Figure 4.11

Nail shedding due to pustular psoriasis.

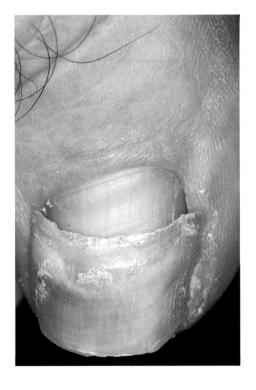

Figure 4.12

Post-traumatic onychomadesis.

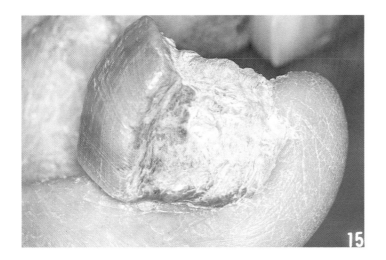

Figure 4.13

Cryptogenic hyperkeratosis.

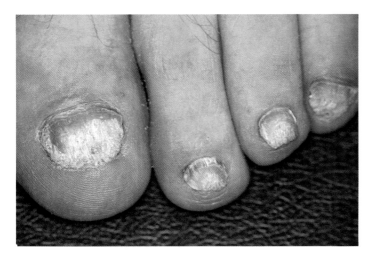

Figure 4.14

Subungual hyperkeratosis due to psoriasis.

Onychogryphosis (Figures 4.16–4.18), a condition mainly seen in the great toe nails of elderly and infirm individuals, is probably due to trauma, footwear pressure, neglect and sometimes associated poor peripheral circulation and fungal infection; these and the less common causes are listed in Table 4.3.

Epithelial hyperplasia of the subungual tissues results from repeated trauma and exudative skin diseases and may occur with

> **If the nail bed is left continuously exposed by nail removal or disease for more than a few months it may produce irregular hyperkeratosis and failure of nail plate adhesion**

any chronic inflammatory condition involving this area. It is especially common in psoriasis, pityriasis rubra pilaris and chronic

Table 4.3 **Causes and associations of onychogryphosis**

Dermatological
Ichthyosis
Psoriasis
Onychomycosis
Syphilis, pemphigus, variola

Local causes
Isolated injury to the nail apparatus
Repeated minor trauma caused by footwear
Foot faults such as hallux valgus

Regional causes
Associated varicose veins
Thrombophlebitis – even in the upper limb
Aneurysms
Elephantiasis
Pathology in the peripheral nervous system

General causes
Old age
Vagrancy and senile dementia
Disease involving the central nervous system
Hyperuricaemia

Idiopathic forms
Acquired or hereditary

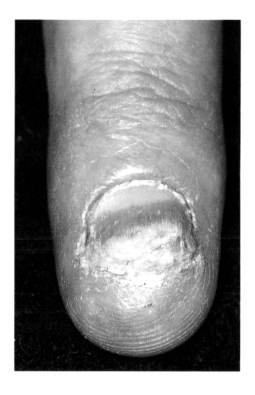

Figure 4.15

Distal subungual hyperkeratosis in psoriasis; note proximal inflammatory brown margin.

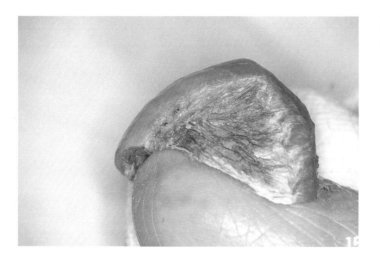

Figure 4.16

Oyster-like onychogryphosis.

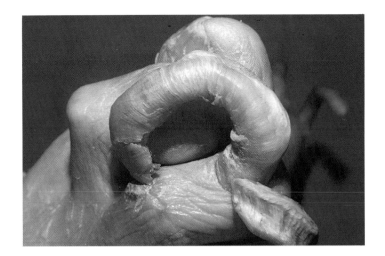

Figure 4.17

Onychogryphosis – ram's horn deformity. (Courtesy of C. Beylot, Bordeaux.)

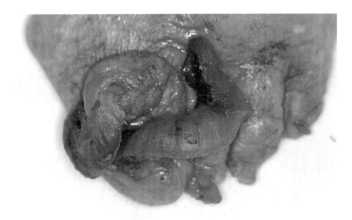

Figure 4.18

Severe onychogryphosis.

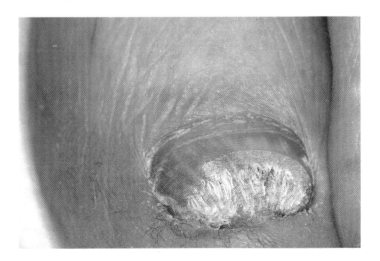

Figure 4.19

Subungual hyperkeratosis due to *Trichophyton rubrum* infection.

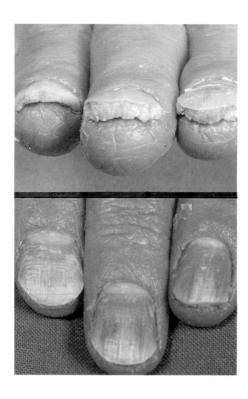

Figure 4.20

Subungual hyperkeratosis due to pityriasis rubra pilaris. (Courtesy of R. Caputo, Milan.)

eczema and may also be due to fungi. Histology reveals periodic acid Schiff reagent (PAS) positive, homogeneous, rounded or oval-shaped, amorphous masses surrounded by normal squamous cells which are usually separated from each other by empty spaces caused by the fixation process. These clumps, which coalesce and enlarge, have been described in psoriasis of the nail, onychomycosis, eczema and alopecia areata and also in some hyperkeratotic processes such as subungual warts and pincer nails. The horny excrescences of the nail bed are not very obvious, but the ridged structure

Table 4.4   **Causes of thick nails (often associated with onycholysis)**

Psoriasis/Reiter's syndrome (Figures 4.14, 4.15)
Onychomycosis (Figure 4.19)
Pityriasis rubra pilaris (PRP) (Figure 4.20)
Pachyonychia congenita (Figures 4.21–4.23)
Contact eczema
   Mineral oils
   Cement workers
   Hair stylists
Acrokeratosis paraneoplastica (Bazex)
Lichen planus
Yellow nail syndrome

Table 4.5   **Causes of thick nails and/or subungual hyperkeratosis**

Frequent
   Onychomycosis (Figure 4.19)
   Psoriasis (Figures 4.14–4.15)
   Contact eczema
      Mineral oils
      Cement workers
      Hair stylists
   Repeated microtrauma
   Single major trauma
   Subungual clavus

Less frequent
   Bowen's disease
   Lichen planus (Figure 4.24)
   Norwegian scabies
   Pachyonychia congenita (Figures 4.21–4.23)
   Pityriasis rubra pilaris (Figure 4.20)
   Bazex's acrokeratosis paraneoplastica
   Reiter's syndrome
   Darier's disease (Figure 4.25)
   Erythroderma
   Ichthyosis
Rare
   Alopecia areata
   Radiodermatitis
   Arsenic keratosis

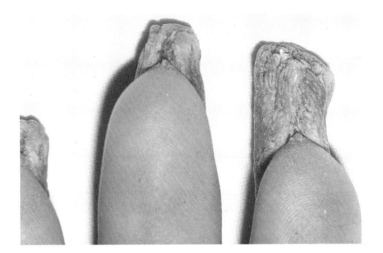

Figure 4.21

Hypertrophic, hard nail in pachyonychia congenita. (Courtesy of Dr Cho, Seoul.)

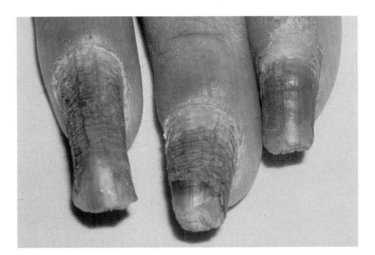

Figure 4.22

Pachyonychia congenita. (Courtesy of Dr Cho, Seoul.)

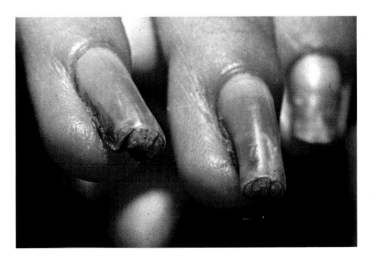

Figure 4.23

Pachyonychia congenita – marked distal subungual thickening. (Courtesy of C. Beylot, Bordeaux.)

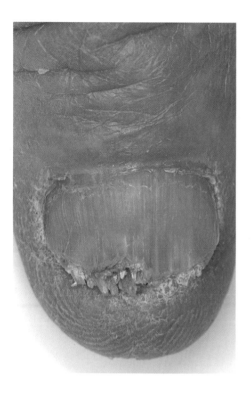

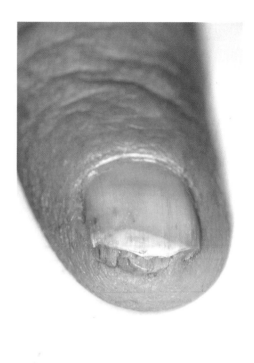

Figure 4.24

Subungual hyperkeratosis due to lichen planus.

Figure 4.25

Darier's disease – distal, irregular, subungual thickening.

may become apparent if the nail plate is cut and shortened.

In keratosis cristarum the keratinizing process is limited to the peripheral area of the nail bed. It starts at its distal portion but may progress somewhat proximally. Scopulariopsis (acaulis) brevicaulis onychomycosis may present with similar changes.

Table 4.4 lists the causes of thick nails often associated with onycholysis; Table 4.5 lists the causes of thick nails and/or subungual hyperkeratosis.

Splinter haemorrhages and subungual haematoma

Splinter haemorrhages

The subungual epidermal ridges extend from the lunula distally to the hyponychium and fit 'tongue-and-groove' fashion between similarly arranged dermal ridges. The disruption of the fine capillaries along these longitudinal dermal ridges results in splinter haemorrhages (Figures 4.26–4.29).

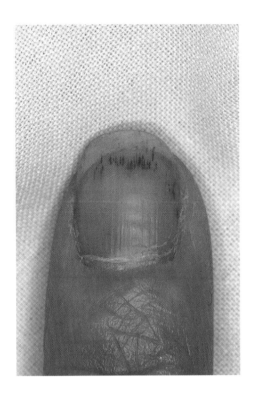

Figure 4.26

Splinter haemorrhages.

Macroscopically, splinter haemorrhages appear as tiny linear structures, usually no greater than 2–3 mm long, arranged in the long axis of the nail. The majority originate within the distal one-third of the nail from the special, 'spirally wound' capillary which produces the pink line normally seen through the nail about 4 mm proximal to the tip of the finger. When the splinter haemorrages originate from the proximal portion of the nail accompanied by a longitudinal xanthonychia, the diagnosis of onychomatri coma should be considered.

The whole nail bed is rarely involved by splinter haemorrhages. When first formed they are plum-coloured but darken to brown or black within 1 to 2 days; subsequently they move superficially and distally with the growth of the nail; at this stage they can be scraped from the undersurface of the nail plate.

The nature of splinter haemorrhages is not clearly known. They may result from emboli in the terminal vessels of the nail bed; the emboli may be septic, or due to trauma of various types; they are commoner in the first three fingers of both hands and develop at the

Figure 4.27

Psoriatic distal subungual splinter haemorrhages.

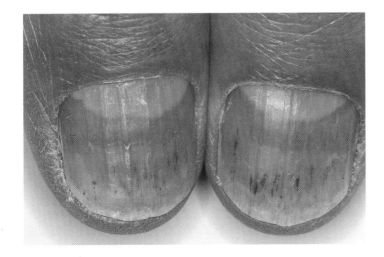

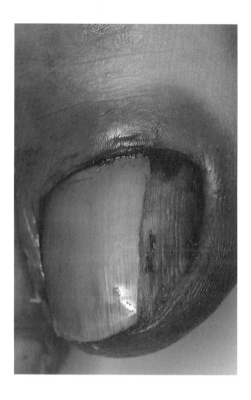

line of separation of the nail plate from the nail bed. Familial capillary fragility may cause splinter haemorrhages in otherwise healthy individuals. Occasional ones are of no clinical significance and are probably traumatic. There is a statistically greater incidence of splinter haemorrhages in males compared to females, and in Negroes compared to white individuals. In healthy females they are usually confined to a single digit.

Histochemical studies of nail parings confirm that the linear discoloration is derived from blood. The blood pigments give a negative Prussian blue and Pearls' reaction.

Many conditions may be associated with splinter haemorrhages (see Table 4.6). In all cases it is probable that, whatever the pathogenesis, the nail bed capillaries are more susceptible to minor trauma leading to linear haemorrhages.

Figure 4.28

Sites of splinter haemorrhages in the nail bed.

Haematomas (see Chapter 9)

Small haemorrhages originating in the nail bed remain subungual as growth progresses

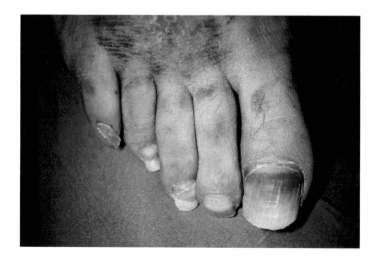

Figure 4.29

Subungual haemorrhage in vitamin C deficiency – scurvy. (Courtesy J.J. Grob, Marseilles)

Table 4.6 Causes of splinter haemorrhages

Amyloidosis
Antiphospholipid syndrome
Arterial emboli
Arthritis (notably rheumatoid arthritis and
  rheumatic fever)
Behçet's disease
Blood dyscrasias (severe anaemia, high altitudes
  purpura)
Buerger's disease
Cirrhosis
Collagen vascular disease
Cryoglobulinaemia (with purpura)
Darier's disease
Drug reactions (especially tetracyclines)
Eczema
Haemochromatosis
Haemodialysis and peritoneal dialysis
Heart disease (notably uncomplicated mitral
  stenosis and subacute bacterial endocarditis)
High-altitude living
Histiocytosis-X
Hypertension
Hypoparathyroidism
Idiopathic (probably traumatic) – up to 20% of
  normal population
Indwelling brachial artery cannula
Malignant neoplasia
Occupational hazards
Onychomatricoma
Onychomycosis
Palmoplantar keratoderma
Peptic ulcer
Pityriasis rubra pilaris
Psoriasis
Pterygium
Pulmonary disease
Radial artery puncture
Raynaud's disease
Renal disease
Sarcoidosis
Scurvy
Septicaemia
Severe illness
Thyrotoxicosis
Minor and repeated trauma
Trichinosis
Vasculitis

distally. The deeper layers of the nail are stained by small pockets of dried blood entrapped in the nail plate. Those produced by trauma to the more proximal part of the matrix will appear in the upper layers of the plate. Sometimes patches of leukonychia overlay haematoma. Moderate trauma to the nail area, or blood dyscrasias, affecting extensive numbers of dermal ridges, determine whether the haemorrhages are punctate or result in large ecchymoses. Acute subungual haematomas are usually obvious, occurring shortly after trauma involving finger or toe nails. The blood which accumulates beneath the nail plate produces pain which may be severe.

Traumatic subungual toe nail haemorrhage may be entirely painless

The technique used for drainage depends on the size and site of the haematoma. Treatment is required to prevent both unnecessary delay in the regrowth of the nail plate and secondary dystrophy which might result from pressure on the matrix due to accumulated blood under the nail.

In acute haematoma of the proximal nail area, drainage of the haematoma with a fine-point scalpel blade or by drilling a hole through the plate will give prompt relief from pain. Hot paper clip cautery is a useful alternative to trephining the plate. This allows blood to be evacuated; the nail is then pressed against the bed by a moderately tight bandage, helping the nail plate to readhere. If this procedure is not immediately practicable, the pain can be relieved by elevating the hand and maintaining the position for approximately 30 minutes.

Occasionally subungual haematoma persists under the nail and does not migrate. A reddish-blue colour, irregular shape, and the absence of colour in the nail plate help to differentiate non-migrating subungual

haematomas from naevi and other causes of
nail pigmentation. It is advisable to remove
the part overlying the subungual haematoma
and identify and remove the old dried blood
in order to establish the diagnosis and to
exclude more significant pathology such as
malignant melanoma.

In total haematoma, often observed when
there is injury to the nail bed, the possibility of an underlying fracture must be considered: X-ray is therefore necessary. The nail is
removed, the haematoma evacuated and the
wound repaired, if necessary with precise
suturing of the nail bed, using 6–0 Dexon or
PDS 6–0. The plate is then cleaned, shortened, narrowed and held in place by suturing
to the lateral nail folds. The stitches are
removed after 10 days, and usually the nail
remains firmly attached.

The differential diagnosis of subungual
blood from melanin may be difficult. As
mentioned above, the haemorrhage is
between the nail plate and the matrix and
nail bed epithelium and gets entrapped by
the regrowing nail. The blood is not therefore degraded to haemosiderin by macro-
phages and is not Prussian blue positive. It
can, however, easily be demonstrated: a
small amount of the pigmented material is
scraped from the nail plate undersurface,
collected in a test tube, a few drops of water
are added and a haemostix is dipped into it.
Due to the pseudo-peroxidase activity of
haemoglobin, the test will be positive
proving the presence of blood.

Subungual bleeding may be due to many
systemic conditions; Table 4.7 lists the
commonest morphological types.

Dorsal and ventral pterygium

Dorsal pterygium consists of a gradual extension of the proximal nail fold over the nail
plate (Figures 4.30–4.32). The nail plate

Table 4.7 Splinter haemorrhages and subungual haematoma in some systemic conditions

	Haematoma	Splinters
Arterial lines/puncture	–	+
Bacterial endocarditis	–	+
Blood dyscrasia	+	+
Cirrhosis	–	+
Collagen vascular disease	+	+
Cryoglobulinaemia	–	+
Drugs	–	+
Dialysis	–	+
Emboli	+	+
Histiocytosis-X (Langerhans cell histiocytosis)	–	+
Scurvy	+	+
Sepsis	–	+
Thyroid	–	+
Vasculitis	–	+

Pterygium is a wing-shaped scar and always irreversible

becomes fissured because of the fusion of the
proximal nail fold epidermis to the nail bed;
its split portions progressively decrease in
size as the pterygium widens. This often
results in two small nail remnants if the
pterygium process is central. Complete
involvement of the matrix and nail bed in
the pathological process leads to total loss of
the nail plate, with permanent atrophy and
scarring in the nail area (see onychatrophy,
page 42). Dorsal pterygium is particularly
seen in scarring lichen planus, less often in

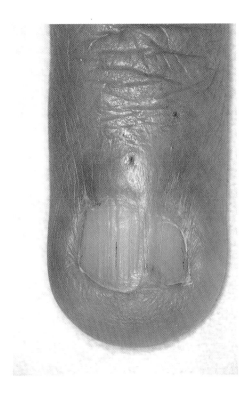

Figure 4.30

Early pterygium scarring in lichen planus.

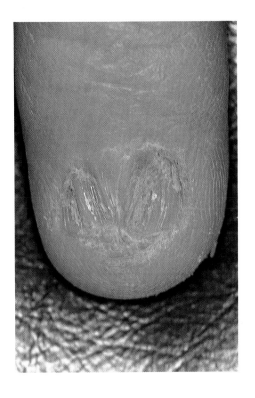

Figure 4.31

Pterygium.

peripheral ischaemia, severe bullous dermatoses, and radiotherapy on the hands of radiologists: it may follow injury; rarely congenital forms occur.

Ventral pterygium, or pterygium inversum unguis (Figure 4.33), is a distal extension of the hyponychial tissue which anchors to the undersurface of the nail, thereby eliminating the distal groove. Scarring in the vicinity of the distal groove, causing it to be obliterated, may produce secondary pterygium inversum unguis. Ventral pterygium may be seen in scleroderma associated with Raynaud's phenomenon, disseminated lupus erythe-

matosus, and causalgia of the median nerve. The condition may be idiopathic, congenital, and familial or acquired. A congenital, aberrant, painful hyponychium has been described associated with oblique, deep fractures of the nails. There are recent reports of familial forms of the disease. In one case an unusual acquired association of pterygium inversum unguis and lenticular atrophy of the palmar creases was recorded.

Pain in the finger tip from minor trauma and haemorrhages may appear when the distal, subungual area is repeatedly pushed back or the nail cut short. Toe nails are

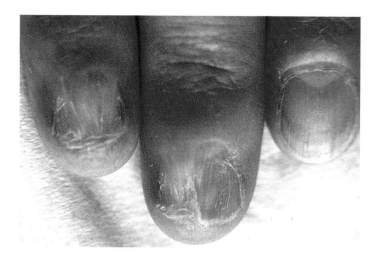

Figure 4.32

Severe pterygium scarring in lichen planus.

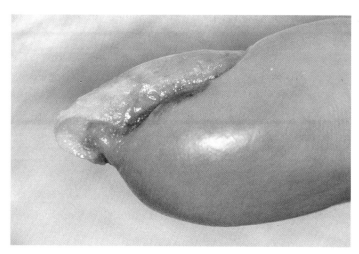

Figure 4.33

Ventral pterygium in acrosclerosis.

only rarely involved. Subungual pterygium (non-inflammatory) is analogous to the claw of lower primates. In patients suffering from dorsal pterygium (excluding the traumatic or congenital types) the main characteristic is dilatation in the nail fold capillary loops and the formation of a slender microvascular shunt system in the more dilated loops. These changes are visible by capillaroscopy.

Table 4.8 lists the well recognized causes of pterygium. Lichen planus is the most common specific cause of dorsal pterygium. Ventral pterygium is most frequently seen in association with Raynaud's disease and systemic sclerosis.

Table 4.8   Causes of pterygium

Dorsal
    Congenital
    Bullous dermatoses (e.g. cicatricial
        pemphigoid,
    Stevens–Johnson syndrome)
    Burns
    Dyskeratosis congenita
    Graft-versus-host disease
    Lichen planus (commonest cause)
    Onychotillomania
    Radiodermatitis
    Raynaud's disease and peripheral vascular
        disease

Ventral
    Congenital
    Familial
    Formaldehyde nail hardeners
    Idiopathic
    Peripheral neuropathy
    Raynaud's disease and systemic sclerosis
    Trauma

Further reading

Achten G, Wanet–Rouard J (1970) Pachyonychia, *Br J Dermatol* **83**: 56–62.

Baran R (1986) Les onycholyses, *Ann Dermatol Vénéréol* **113**: 159–170.

Baran R, Badillet G (1982) Primary onycholysis of the big toenails. A review of 113 cases, *Br J Dermatol* **106**: 526–534.

Baran R, Juhlin L (1987) Drug-induced photoonycholysis. Three subtypes identified in a study of 15 cases, *J Am Acad Dermatol* **17**: 1012–1016.

Caputo R, Cappio F, Rigon C *et al* (1993) Pterygium inversum unguis. Report of 19 cases and review of the literature, *Arch Dermatol* **129**: 1307–1309.

DePaoli RT, Marks VJ (1987) Crusted (Norwegian) scabies: treatment of nail involvement, *J Am Acad Dermatol*, **17**: 136–138.

Kechijian P (1985) Onycholysis of the fingernails: evaluation and management, *J Am Acad Dermatol* **12**: 552–560.

Ray L (1963) Onycholysis, *Arch Dermatol Syphil* **88**: 181.

Runne V, Orfanos Ce (1981) The human nail, *Curr Prob Dermatol* **9**: 102–149.

Sonnex TS, Dawber RPR, Zachary CB *et al* (1986) The nails in type I pityriasis rubra pilaris: a comparison with Sézary syndrome and psoriasis, *J Am Acad Dermatol*, **15**: 956–960.

5 Periungual tissue disorders

Paronychia

The proximal nail fold (PNF), with its distal cuticle attached to the nail and the ventral eponychium, is normally well adapted to prevent infections and external inflammatory agents entering the proximal matrix area; the same is true of the lateral nail walls and folds. It is therefore probable that no paronychia is truly primary, there always being some physical or chemical damage preceding the infection or inflammation; this is less true in relation to superficial infections on the dorsum of the PNF, such as the so-called bulla repens (a bullous form of impetigo).

Acute paronychia

> **Acute paronychia needs urgent systemic antibiotic treatment to avoid permanent nail dystrophy**

Minor trauma is a frequent cause of this infection and surgical treatment may be necessary. Acute paronychia may follow a break in the skin (for example, if a hang nail is torn), a splinter under the distal edge of the nail, a prick from a thorn in a lateral groove or, sometimes, from subungual infection secondary to haematoma (Figures 5.1, 5.2).

The infection begins in the lateral paronychial areas with local redness, swelling and pain. At this stage medical treatment is indicated: wet compresses (for example with Burrow's aluminium acetate solution) and appropriate systemic antibiotic therapy are given. Because the continuation of antibiotics may mask developing pathology which can damage the nail apparatus, if acute paronychia does not show clear signs of response within two days then surgical treatment should be instituted under proximal block local anaesthesia. The purulent reaction may take several days to localize and during this time throbbing pain is always a major symptom. The collection of pus may easily be seen through the nail or at the paronychial fold. Sometimes a bead of pus may be present in the periungual groove. In the absence of visible pus, the gathering gives rise to tension and the lesion should be incised at the site of maximum pain, not necessarily at the site of maximum swelling. In practice, Bunell's technique is usually successful: the base of the nail (the proximal third) is removed by cutting across

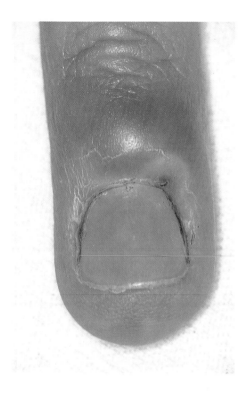

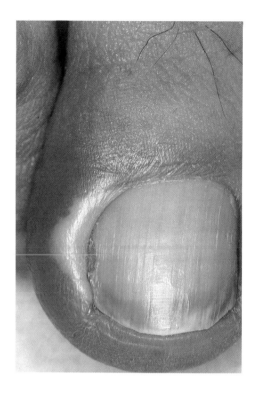

Figure 5.1

Acute bacterial paronychia.

Figure 5.2

Acute bacterial paronychia – pus tracking within
the lateral nail fold.

with pointed scissors. A non-adherent gauze
wick is laid under the proximal nail fold. If the
paronychial infection remains restricted to one
side, removal of the homologous lateral part of
the nail is sufficient.

Bacterial culture and sensitivity studies are
mandatory. The bacteria most commonly
found in acute paronychia are staphylococci
and, less commonly, β-haemolytic streptococci and gram-negative enteric bacteria.
Should surgical intervention be delayed, the
pus will track around the base of the nail
under the proximal nail fold and inflame the
matrix; it may then be responsible for

transient or permanent dystrophy of the nail
plate. It is essential to note that the nail
matrix in early childhood is particularly
fragile and can be destroyed within 48 hours
by acute bacterial infection. The pus may
also separate the nail from its loose, underlying proximal attachment. The firmer
attachment of the nail at the distal border of
the lunula may temporarily limit the spread
of the pus. In cases with extension of the
infection under the distal nail bed, the whole
of the nail base should be removed with nail
removed distally to expose fully the involved
nail bed.

Distal subungual pyogenic infection may or may not be secondary to the periungual varieties. A U-shaped piece of the distal nail plate is excised in the region loosened by the pus and debridement of the affected nail bed carried out. Extension of the infection may involve the finger pulp or the matrix.

Sometimes the evacuation of a perionychial phlyctenular abscess uncovers a narrow sinus; this may be part of a 'collar-stud' abscess which communicates with a deeper, necrotic zone; it must be exposed and excised.

If acute paronychia accompanies ingrowing nail, the treatment must be supplemented by removing all offending portions of the nail plate. After surgery, the dressing is kept moist with saline or an antiseptic soak. This should be changed daily after bathing in antiseptic soap until the purulent discharge stops – preferably with full splinting and immobilization of finger, hand and forearm.

In general, acute paronychia involves only one nail. In chronic or subacute paronychia, which may mimic acute paronychia, several finger nails may be infected. The differential diagnosis includes:

- Paronychial inflammation of the finger nails accompanying chronic eczema.
- Herpes simplex.
- Psoriasis and Reiter's disease, which may also involve the proximal nail fold.
- Acute ischaemia where the finger is cold.

Chronic paronychia

> **Chronic paronychia of the hands is typically initiated by frequent wet activities and occupations**

Chronic paronychia is an inflammatory disorder of the proximal nail fold typically affecting hands which are continually exposed to a wet environment and repeated minor trauma that causes cuticle damage. When the cuticle is torn or lost, the epidermal barrier of the proximal nail fold is impaired and the proximal nail fold is then exposed to a large number of environmental hazards. Irritants and allergens may easily penetrate the proximal nail fold and produce contact dermatitis that is responsible for the chronic inflammation. An immediate hypersensitivity (Type I) reaction to food ingredients is sometimes seen.

The condition is prevalent in people in contact with water, soap, detergents and other chemicals; it is particularly prevalent in housewives. There is also a high incidence among chefs, barmen, confectioners and fishmongers. The index and middle finger of the left hand are most often affected, these being the digits most subject to minor trauma such as rubbing during hand washing of clothes.

Clinically, the proximal and lateral nail folds show erythema and swelling. The cuticle is lost and the ventral portion of the proximal nail fold becomes separated from the nail plate. This newly formed space has an important additional role in maintaining and aggravating chronic paronychia – it becomes a receptacle for micro-organisms and environmental particles that potentiates the chronic inflammation. With time the nail fold retracts and becomes thickened and rounded.

> **Chronic paronychia is not a primary infection**

The course of chronic paronychia is interspersed with self-limiting episodes of painful acute inflammation. The acute exacerbations of chronic paronychia may be due to secondary *Candida* and bacterial infections, with small abscesses resulting at the depth of the space between the proximal nail fold and the nail plate. These microbial abscesses drain spontaneously and this explains why such bacterial exacerbations subside without treatment in a few days.

Acute exacerbations of chronic paronychia are not only due to microbial colonization, but can also be caused by irritants or allergens that penetrate deep to the proximal nail fold. Foreign material such as wax, hair, foodstuffs and debris may collect in the proximal nail fold. This may cause retraction of the nail fold and persistence of the process.

In the early stages the nail plate is unaffected, but one or both lateral edges may develop irregularities and yellow, brown or blackish discoloration; this may extend over a large portion of the nail and occasionally the whole nail may become involved. It is believed to follow discoloration caused by dihydroxyacetone produced by the organisms in the nail fold. By contrast, *Pseudomonas* often produces a greenish discoloration. The lateral discoloured edges of the nail plate become cross-ridged when the disease mainly affects the lateral nail fold. On the surface, which often becomes rough and friable, numerous irregular transverse ridges or waves appear as a result of repeated acute exacerbations. Eventually the size of the nail is considerably reduced, an effect which is exaggerated by the swelling of the surrounding soft tissues. The pathology of chronic paronychia reveals spongiotic dermatitis of the ventral portion of the proximal nail fold.

There is some disagreement as to the importance of yeasts in chronic *Candida* paronychia; this organism may be commensal or pathogenic. The various factors which damage the area allow *Staphylococcus aureus* and *Candida* species to attack the keratin and cause the detachment of the cuticle from the nail plate. In children the most common predisposing factor to chronic *Candida* paronychia is the habit of thumb or finger sucking. This is potentially more harmful than occupational immersion, as saliva is more irritating than water. Paronychia may also develop in patients with eczema or psoriasis involving the nail folds. Although infrequent, chronic paronychia of the toe nails may develop in association with diabetes mellitus or peripheral vascular disease, both of which should be excluded unless ingrowing nail is present.

Differential diagnosis

Chronic paronychia can be associated with nail infections caused by *Scytalidium spp.* Brown discoloration starting at the lateral edges of the nail and spreading centrally into the nail is seen in some cases. Rarely this is caused by separate *Candida* infection which is not directly related to the original *Scytalidium* infection. In white Caucasians, *Fusarium oxysporum* may produce chronic paronychia in finger or toe nails.

Syphilitic paronychia is due to a chancre on the perionychial area; it is usually painful. Pemphigus may produce considerable bolstering of the nail fold and closely resembles chronic paronychia with accompanying onychomycosis. Parakeratosis pustulosa (Hjorth Sabouraud's syndrome) may also mimic fungal paronychia. Psoriatic lesions, Reiter's disease and eczema sometimes involve the proximal nail fold. Secondary bacterial or yeast infections may develop in the area.

If chronic paronychia becomes recalcitrant and unresponsive to medical procedures, then surgical removal of the proximal nail fold and proximal lateral nail folds together with the proximal nail plate may be required; after this procedure complete healing normally takes approximately 8 weeks.

Table 5.1 shows the principal causes of paronychia. Acute paronychia is most commonly seen in nail biters, whilst the most frequently seen type of chronic paronychia is

Table 5.1   Causes of paronychia

Infective
  Acute
    Viral
    Bacterial (Figures 5.1, 5.2)
    Fungal
    Parasitic
  Chronic
    Mycotic (Figure 5.3)
    Myobacterial
    Syphilitic

Drugs
  Retinoids (Figure 5.4)

Cosmetic
  Trauma
  Epoxy resin dermatitis

Occupational

Dermatoses
  Acrodermatitis enteropathica (Figure 5.5)
  Contact dermatitis
  Darier's disease
  Dyskeratosis congenita
  Eczema
  Hallopeau's acrodermatitis
  Ingrowing toe nail (Figure 5.6)
  Lichen planus
  Pachyonychia congenita
  Parakeratosis pustulosa (Figure 5.7)
  Pemphigus
  Psoriasis–Reiter's syndrome (Figure 5.8)
  Radiodermatitis
  Yellow nail syndrome

Systemic disease
  Collagen vascular diseases (Figure 5.9)
  Encephalitis
  Frostbite
  Histiocytosis-X
  Ischaemia (acute)
  Leukaemia
  Metastases
  Neuropathy
  Paraneoplastic acrokeratosis
  Sarcoidosis (Figure 5.10)
  Stevens–Johnson syndrome
  Vasculitis
  Zinc deficiency (Figure 5.11)

Miscellaneous
  Finger-sucking children
  Foreign body granuloma

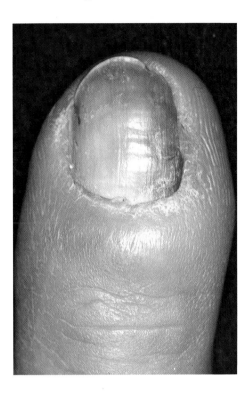

Figure 5.3

Chronic paronychia due to constant wetting.

that occurring on the hands of domestic and office cleaners and bar staff (wet work) (Figure 5.3).

Ragged cuticles and 'hang nail'

Thickened, hyperkeratotic, irregular (ragged) cuticles (Figure 5.12) are most commonly seen in dermatomyositis (Figure 5.13). Perionychial tissues are constantly subjected to trauma. In nail biters and 'pickers' the cuticles and nail folds may show considerable damage, erosions, haemorrhage and

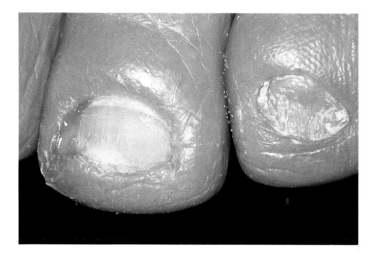

Figure 5.4

Chronic paronychia due to oral etretinate therapy.

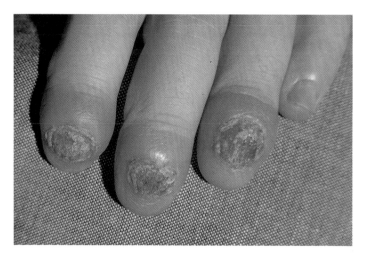

Figure 5.5

Chronic paronychia in acrodermatitis. (Courtesy of Professor Bourlond.)

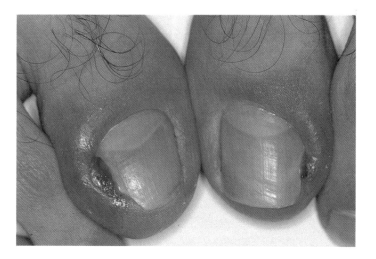

Figure 5.6

Chronic paronychia with granulation tissue due to oral isotretinoin therapy.

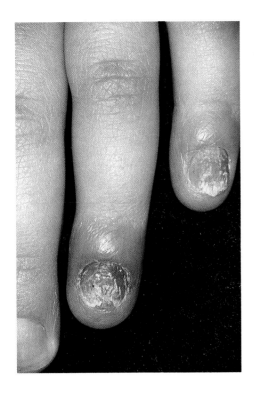

Figure 5.7

Chronic paronychia in psoriasis.

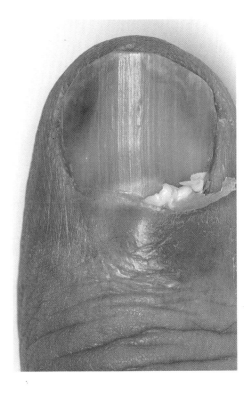

Figure 5.8

Chronic paronychia in psoriasis.

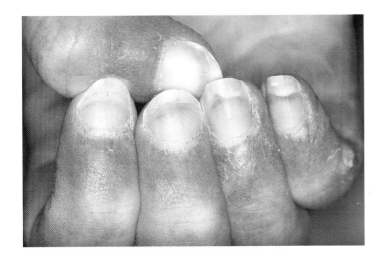

Figure 5.9

Paronychial inflammation due to systemic lupus erythematosus.

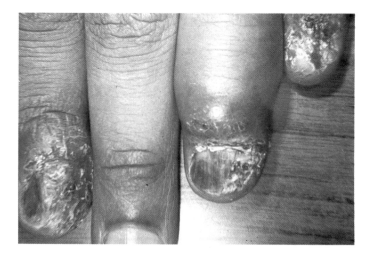

Figure 5.10

Chronic granulomatous paronychia due to sarcoidosis. (Courtesy of J. Hewitt.)

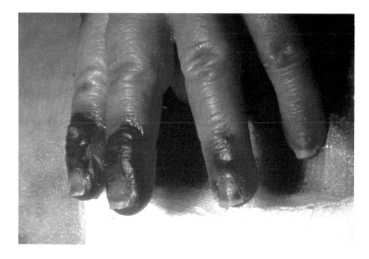

Figure 5.11

Paronychia due to zinc deficiency.

crusting. The ulnar side of the nail fold and cuticle is most vulnerable and there may be small triangular tags of skin (hang nail, Figure 5.14) and separated spicules of nail, still attached proximally. Thickened cuticule composed of several layers (onion-like) can be an unusual manifestation of factitious damage.

Hang nails may also result from occupational injuries, due to the hydration and dehydration caused by frequent wetting. However, usually hang nail has no obvious cause, though it may be self-induced.

Painful dorsolateral fissures of the finger tip

In subjects with dry skin, particularly in winter, painful dorsolateral fissures may be

(a)

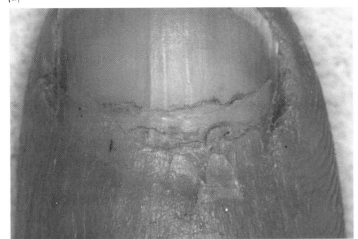

(b)

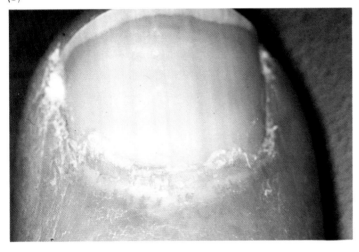

Figure 5.12

Ragged cuticles: (a) unknown cause; (b) scleroderma.

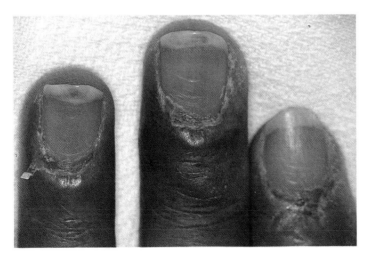

Figure 5.13

Dermatomyositis with ragged cuticles.

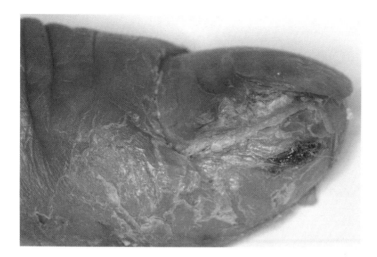

Figure 5.14

'Hang nail' deformity of the lateral nail.

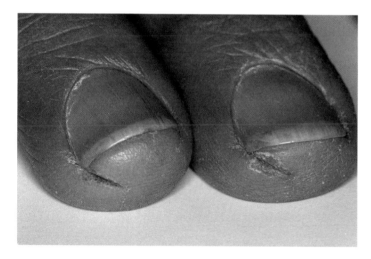

Figure 5.15

Dorsolateral fissures – usually very painful.

seen located distal to the lateral nail groove (Figure 5.15). This appears to be a sign of atopy.

Tumours and swellings

Table 5.2 lists some of the commoner lesions in relation to their site in the nail apparatus.

Benign and malignant lesions are detailed in Table 5.3. The nail apparatus develops *in utero* from primitive skin and it is therefore not surprising that many of the swellings and tumours that affect the rest of the skin can occur within it. Table 5.4 lists the vast array of such conditions which have been described in and around the nail apparatus; only the distinctive lesions which are peculiar to the nail apparatus and those

Table 5.2   Tumours of the nail unit (by site)

At the nail fold/plate junction
  Acquired periungual fibrokeratoma
  Periungual fibroma (tuberous sclerosis)

Within the nail fold
  Myxoid pseudocysts
  Tendon sheath giant cell tumour
  Verruca vulgaris

Within the nail bed with or without nail plate destruction
  Subungual exostosis
  Osteochondroma
  Enchondroma
  Subungual corn (heloma)
  Pyogenic granuloma
  Glomus tumour
  Recurring digital fibrous tumour of childhood
  Bowen's disease and squamous cell carcinoma
  Melanoma
  Metastases

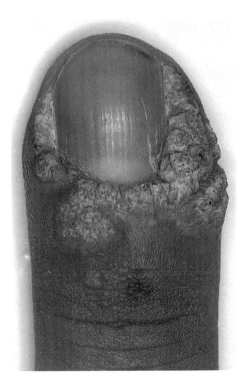

Figure 5.16

Periungual viral warts.

which have different morphology in this site will be described in detail.

Periungual and subungual warts

Common warts are caused by human papilloma viruses of different biological types (Figures 5.16–5.18). They are benign, weakly infective, fibro-epithelial tumours with a rough keratotic surface. Usually periungual warts are asymptomatic, although fissuring may cause pain. Subungual warts initially affect the hyponychium, growing slowly toward the nail bed and finally elevating the nail plate. Bone erosion from verruca vulgaris occasionally occurs, although some of these cases may have been keratocanthomas since the latter, epidermoid carcinoma and verruca vulgaris are sometimes indistinguishable by clinical signs alone.

Subungual warts are painful and may mimic glomus tumour. The nail plate is not often affected, but surface ridging may occur and, more rarely, dislocation of the nail. Biting, picking and tearing of the nail and nail walls are common habits in subjects with periungual warts. This type of trauma is responsible for the spread of warts and their resistance to treatment.

Tuberculosis cutis verrucosa (butcher's nodule) may rarely pose differential diagnostic problems, but it is very rare in the periungual location, affecting a lateral fold of the toe nails with long-standing warty lesions

Table 5.3 Differential diagnosis of subungual malignant melanoma

Malignant lesions	Benign lesions
Pigmented	LM
Haemangioendothelioma	Melanocytic hyperplasia
Kaposi's sarcoma	Junctional naevus
Metastatic melanoma	Adrenal insufficiency
	Adrenalectomy for Cushing's disease
	Angiokeratoma
	Chromogenic bacteria (*Proteus*)
	Drugs: antimalarials, cytotoxics, arsenic, silver, thallium, phenothiazines and PUVA
	Haematoma, trauma
	Irradiation
	Laugier–Hunziker–Baran syndrome
	Onychomycosis nigricans
Amelanotic	
Basal cell carcinoma	Epidermal cyst
Bowen's disease	Exostosis
Squamous cell carcinoma	Foreign body granuloma
Metastasis	Keratoacanthoma
	Pyogenic granuloma
	Ingrowing nail

with unusual wart morphology. Bowen's disease must be considered, as should the subcutaneous vegetations of systemic amyloidosis.

Treatment of periungual warts is often frustrating. X-ray and radium treatment has become obsolete. Saturated monochloro-acetic acid has been suggested but is painful; it is applied sparingly, allowed to dry and then covered with 40% salicylic acid plaster cut to the size of the wart and held in place with adhesive tape for 2 to 3 days. After 1 to 2 weeks many of the warts can be removed and the procedure repeated. Subungual warts are treated similarly, after cutting away the overlying part of the nail plate. Recalcitrant warts may respond to weekly applications of diphencyprone solutions ranging from 0.2 to 2%, according to the patient's ability to produce a good inflammatory reaction. Some authorities recommend the use of canthari-din (0.07%); this is applied to the lesions and covered by a plastic tape for 24 hours. The resultant blister should be retreated at 2 week intervals, three to four times if neces-sary. Recent work strongly recommends

Table 5.4   **Range of tumours and swellings affecting the nail apparatus (Those underlined are described in the text)**

Warts
Verrucous epidermal naevus
Subungual papilloma
Verrucous lesions in incontinentia pigmenti
Subungual corn
Epidermoid cyst
Fibromata
    Keloids
    Dermatofibroma
    Koenen's tumour
    Acquired periungual fibrokeratoma
    Subungual filamentous tumour
    Benign juvenile digital fibromatosis
Leiomyoma
Giant cell tumour
Xanthoma
Lipoma
Neurogenic tumours
Multicentric reticulohistocytosis
Actinic keratosis
Arsenical keratosis
Glomus tumour
Pyogenic granuloma
Naevus flammeus and angioma
Angiokeratoma circumscriptum
Aneurysmal bone cyst (arteriovenous fistula)
Subungual exostosis
Enchondroma
    Maffucci's syndrome
Osteoid osteoma
Hereditary multiple exostosis (diaphysial
    aclasis)
Myxoid pseudocyst
Myxoma
Bowen's disease
Squamous cell carcinoma
Keratoacanthoma
Basal cell carcinoma
Sarcoma
Kaposi's sarcoma
Lymphoma
Metastases
Melanotic/melanocytic lesions
    Benign melanocytic hyperplasia
    Lentigo simplex and naevocytic naevus
    Atypical melanocytic hyperplasia
    Peutz–Jeghers–Touraine syndrome
    Malignant melanoma
    Laugier–Hunziker–Baran syndrome

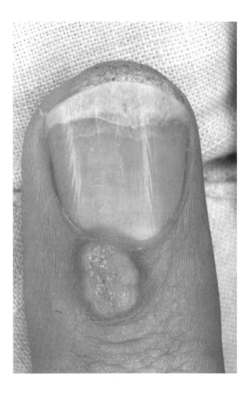

Figure 5.17

Proximal nail fold viral wart with associated nail plate depression.

bleomycin for recalcitrant warts; it is given intralesionally 1 µg per ml at 2 week intervals. Some patients find this more painful than correctly used cryosurgery!

Surgical treatment should be avoided if possible. Cryosurgery with carbon dioxide snow or liquid nitrogen is often used but may cause blistering, with the blister roof containing the epidermal wart component if the treatment succeeds. However, when treating the proximal nail fold freezing must not be prolonged since the matrix may easily be damaged; this may result in circumscribed leukonychia or even nail dystrophy, although

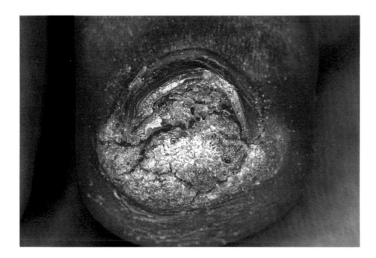

Figure 5.18

Viral wart distorting the nail plate and nail bed. (Courtesy of G. Cannata.)

scarring is rare with cryosurgery. Particular side-effects of cryosurgery include pain, depigmentation and secondary bacterial infection (rare), Beau's lines, onychomadesis, nail loss or inordinate oedema, the latter often worse in the very young and very old, and transient neuropathy or anaesthesia. Many of the side-effects are avoidable if the freezing times used are carefully controlled and if prophylactic analgesic and subsequent anti-inflammatory treatment is carried out – soluble aspirin 600 mg three times daily for 5 days and topical steroid application twice daily. Destruction by curettage and electrodesiccation may produce considerable scarring. Infra red coagulation and argon and carbon dioxide laser treatments have been used recently with some success. If the most aggressive measures fail, or compliance is poor, formalin may be applied daily with a wooden toothpick. If the lesions become inflamed, fissured or tender, because of the therapy or secondary infection, treatment is interrupted and a topical antiseptic preparation used for several days.

Many lay and medical people have 'tricks' for attempting to cure warts, such as 'wrapping', followed 2 weeks later by the careful application of liquified phenol, then a drop of nitric acid to the lesion. The fuming and spluttering that occurs looks efficaceous and the wart turns brown!

Since the incubation period of human warts may be up to several months, consistent follow-up, even after seemingly successful therapy, is necessary to allow for early treatment of newly growing warts.

Fibromas

Many different types of fibromas may occur in and around the nail (Figure 5.19). They may be true entities or merely variants of one process.

Keloids

Hypertrophic scars and keloids result from injuries to the nail fold or nail bed and may significantly distort the nail apparatus.

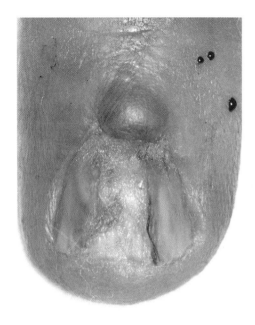

Figure 5.19

Periungual fibroma.

Dermatofibromas

Nail apparatus dermatofibromas are rare and may resemble cutaneous horns, fibrokeratomas or supernumerary digits; the latter, however, usually arise on the ulnar aspect of the fifth metacarpophalangeal joint. The histological changes include areas of very thick, hypocellular, hyalinized collagen bundles, randomly orientated; there is an ill defined nodule situated mainly in the reticular dermis; elastic fibres are often scarce or absent.

Koenen's tumour

Koenen's periungual fibromas develop in 50% of cases of tuberous sclerosis (epiloia or Bourneville–Pringle disease). They usually appear at about 12–14 years of age and increase progressively in size and number with age. Individual tumours are small, round, flesh coloured and asymptomatic, with a smooth surface (Figures 5.20, 5.21). The tip may be slightly hyperkeratotic, resembling fibrokeratoma. They grow out from the nail fold, eventually overgrowing the nail bed and destroying the nail plate. Depending on their site of origin, they may cause longitudinal depressions in the nail plate. Excessively large tumours are often painful, requiring excision. Histological changes consist of dense angiofibrotic tissue, sometimes with neuroglial tissue at the centre, and hyperkeratosis at the tip.

Koenen's tumours are cured by simple excision. Usually no suture is necessary. Tumours growing out from under the proximal nail fold are removed after reflecting the proximal nail fold back by making lateral incisions down each margin in the axis of the lateral nail grooves. Subungual fibromas are removed after avulsion of the corresponding part of the nail plate.

Acquired periungual fibrokeratoma

Acquired periungual fibrokeratomas are probably identical to acquired digital fibrokeratomas and Steel's garlic clove fibroma. They are acquired, benign, spontaneously developing, asymptomatic nodules with a hyperkeratotic tip and a narrow base (Figures 5.22, 5.23). They most commonly occur in the periungual area or on other parts of the fingers. A case was described in which the lesion was located beneath the nail, visible under the free margin of the great toe nail. Most periungual fibrokeratomas emerge from the most proximal part of the nail sulcus

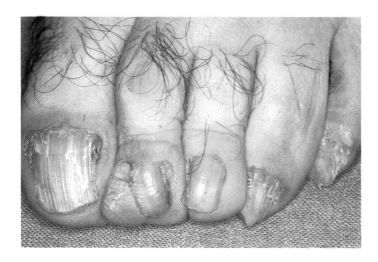

Figure 5.20

Koenen's tumours (tuberous sclerosis). (Courtesy of C. Beylot, Bordeaux.)

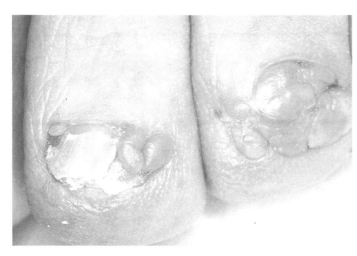

Figure 5.21

Multiple Koenen's tumours.

growing on the nail and causing a sharp longitudinal depression. Trauma is thought to be a major factor initiating acquired periungual fibrokeratoma.

Microscopically, acquired periungual fibrokeratomas resemble hyperkeratotic 'dermal herniae'. The core consists of mature eosinophilic collagen fibres orientated along the main vertical axis of the tumour. The connective tissue cells are increased. Most fibromas are highly vascular. The epidermis is thick and acanthotic. There is a marked orthokeratotic horny layer, which may be parakeratotic and contains serum or blood at the tip of the tumour. Elastic fibres are normal. Acid mucopolysaccharides are not increased.

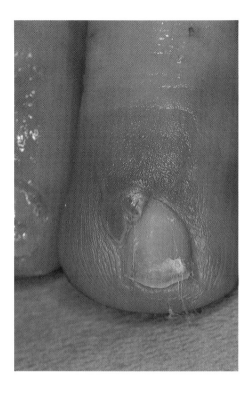

Figure 5.22

Acquired fibrokeratoma.

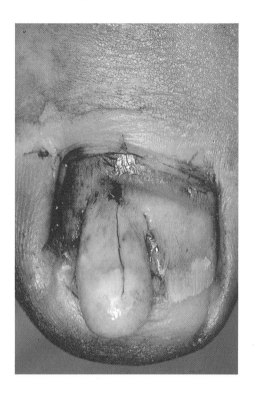

Figure 5.23

'Garlic clove' fibrokeratoma.

Surgical treatment is the same as for Koenen's tumours and depends on the size and location of the lesion.

The differential diagnosis of acquired periungual fibroma includes:

- Keloid
- Koenen's tumour
- Recurring digital fibrous tumours of childhood
- Dermatofibrosarcoma
- Fibrosarcoma
- Acrochordon
- Cutaneous horn

- Eccrine poroma
- Pyogenic granuloma
- Verruca vulgaris and
- Exostosis.

Subungual filamentous tumour

Subungual filamentous tumours are thread-like, horny, subungual lesions growing with the nail plate and emerging from under the free edge of it. They may cause a longitudinal rim. This entity is probably a narrow, extremely hyperkeratotic fibrokeratoma; it can be pared down painlessly when the nail is cut.

Recurring digital fibrous tumours of childhood (benign juvenile digital fibromatosis)

Recurring digital fibrous tumours (RDFT) are round, smooth, firm tumours with a reddish or livid-red colour. They are located on the dorsal and axial surfaces of the fingers and toes, characteristically sparing the thumbs and great toes (Figure 5.24). They may present at birth or develop during infancy, although one single case was recently described in an adult. There is no sex predominance. Fingers are more often affected than toes. On reaching the nail unit, they may elevate the nail plate, leading to dystrophy but not to destruction. Often the tumour is multicentric, occurring on several digits. Although an infectious origin is probable, no virus has been isolated and viral particles have not been demonstrated by electron microscopy. Up to 60% recur after excision. Spontaneous regression was noted in 5 out of 61 cases; regression may be hastened by cryosurgery. Radical surgical ablation of the area involved may rarely be necessary, including the nail unit, leading to permanent loss of the nail. Firm plantar nodules may be associated with these tumours.

Histology shows a diffuse, proliferative, cellular process in the dermis with increased numbers of apparently normal fibroblasts with uniform, spindle-shaped nuclei. Mitoses are absent or rare. Elastic tissue is decreased. In about 2% of the fibroblasts, paranuclear inclusion bodies, 3 to 10 µm in diameter, can be seen in adequately fixed specimens using stains such as iron haematoxylin, methyl green–pyronin and phosphotungstic acid–haematoxylin. Electron microscopy shows that the inclusions consist of fibrillar masses without a limiting membrane. On the basis of

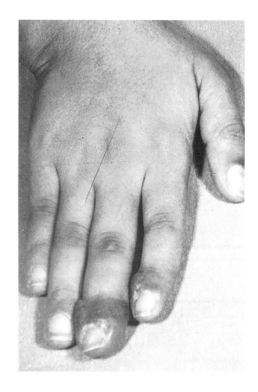

Figure 5.24

Juvenile fibromatosis.

this evidence, it has been suggested that the condition should be termed 'elastodysplasia'.

Glomus tumour

The glomus tumour was first described almost 200 years ago as a painful, subcutaneous 'tubercle'. Several cases were described as malignant angiosarcomas or colloid sarcomas. Seventy-five per cent of glomus tumours occur in the hand, especially in the fingertips and particularly the subungual

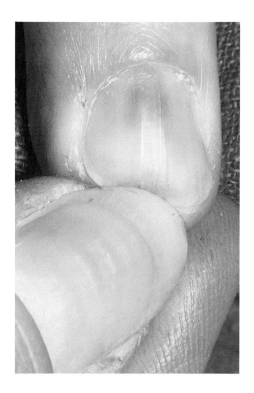

Figure 5.25

Glomus tumour.

millimetres in diameter, rarely exceeding 1 cm in diameter (Figure 5.25). Sometimes it causes a slight rise in surface temperature which can be detected by thermography. Minor nail deformities are caused by 50% of the tumours – ridging or a nail plate 'gutter' being the commonest. A similar proportion cause a depression on the dorsal aspect of the distal phalangeal bone or even a cyst visible on X-ray. Probing, which elicits pain, and transillumination may help to localize the tumour if it is not clearly visible through the nail. If the tumour cannot be localized clinically or on X-ray, arteriography should be performed; this will reveal a star-shaped telangiectatic zone. In selected cases, MRI has been shown to help in the diagnosis of a glomus tumour of the finger tip, revealing even very small lesions.

Many patients give a history of trauma. The most common misdiagnoses are neuroma, causalgia, gout and arthritis. Histology shows a highly differentiated, organoid tumour. It consists of an afferent arteriole, vascular channels lined with endothelium and surrounded by irregularly arranged cuboidal cells with round dark nuclei and pale cytoplasm. Primary collecting veins drain into the cutaneous veins. Myelinated and non-myelinated nerves are found and may account for the pain. The tumour is surrounded by a fibrous capsule. Since all the elements of the normal glomus are present, the glomus tumour may be considered as a hamartoma rather than a true tumour.

Treatment is by surgical excision. Small tumours may be removed by punching a 6 mm hole in the nail plate, incising the nail bed and enucleating the lesion. The small nail disc is put back in its original position as a physiological dressing. Larger tumours may be treated after removal of the proximal half of the nail plate; those in lateral positions are removed by an L-shaped incision parallel to and 4 to 6 mm on the volar side of the lateral nail fold. The nail bed is carefully dissected from the bone until

area. Between 1 and 2% of all hand tumours are glomus tumours. The age at the time of diagnosis ranges from 30 to 50 years. Men are less frequently affected than women.

The tumour is characterized by intense, often pulsating pain that may be spontaneous or provoked by the slightest trauma. Even changes in temperature, especially from warm to cold, may trigger pain radiating up to the shoulder. Sometimes the pain is worse at night: it may disappear when a tourniquet is applied.

The tumour is seen through the nail plate as a small, bluish to reddish-blue spot several the tumour is reached and removed. This is usually curative, although the pain may take several weeks to disappear. Recurrences occur in 10–20% of cases and may represent either incomplete excision or adjacent tumours overlooked at the initial operation, or genuine new growth. More extensive surgery than is often carried out might achieve more first time cures.

Subungual exostosis

> **Distorted nail shape may be due to bone tumours**

Subungual exostoses are not true tumours but rather outgrowths of normal bone or calcified cartilaginous remains (Figures 5.26a–c). Whether or not subungual osteochondroma is a different entity is not clear.

Subungual exostoses are painful bony growths which elevate the nail. They are particularly frequent in young people and are mostly located in the great toe, although less commonly subungual exostoses also occur on the fingers. They start as small elevations of the dorsal aspect of the distal phalanx and eventually emerge from under the nail edge or destroy the nail plate. If the nail is shed, the surface becomes eroded and secondarily infected, sometimes mimicking ingrown toe nail. Walking may be painful.

Trauma appears to be a major causative factor, although some authors claim that a history of trauma only occurs in a minority. The triad of pain (the leading symptom), nail deformation and radiographic features is usually diagnostic. The exostosis is a trabeculated osseous growth with an expanded distal portion covered with radiolucent fibrocartilage.

Osteochondroma, commonly presenting with the same symptoms, has a male predominance. There is often a history of trauma. Its growth rate is slow. X-ray examination shows a well defined, sessile, bony growth with a hyaline cartilage cap which must be differentiated from primary subungual calcification; the latter is particularly seen in older women, and secondary subungual calcification due to trauma and psoriasis.

Treatment is by excision of the excess bone under full aseptic conditions. The nail plate is partially removed and a longitudinal incision made in the nail bed. The osseous growth with its cartilaginous cap is carefully dissected, using fine skin hooks to avoid damage to the fragile nail bed. The tumour is removed with a fine chisel but, whenever possible, the tumour should be removed by an L-shaped or 'fish mouth' incision, in order to avoid avulsion of the nail plate.

Myxoid pseudocysts of the digits

The many synonyms for this lesion reflect its controversial nature:

- Dorsal finger cyst
- Synovial cyst
- Recurring myxomatous cyst
- Cutaneous myxoid cyst
- Dorsal distal interphalangeal joint ganglion
- Digital mucinous pseudocyst
- Focal myxomatous degeneration
- Mucoid cyst.

Whereas some authors regard it as a synovial cyst, most now believe it to be a periarticular degenerative lesion.

Myxoid cysts occur more often in women. They are typically found in the proximal nail fold of the fingers and rarely on toes (Figures 5.27–5.29). Usually asymptomatic, they vary from soft to firm, cystic to fluctuant, and may be dimpled, dome-shaped or smooth-surfaced. Transillumination confirms their cystic nature. They are always located to one

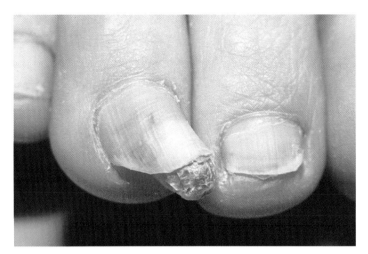

(a)

Figure 5.26

(a,b) Exostosis; (c) X-ray of (b).

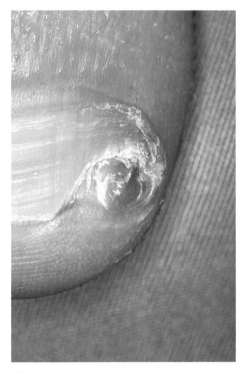

(b)

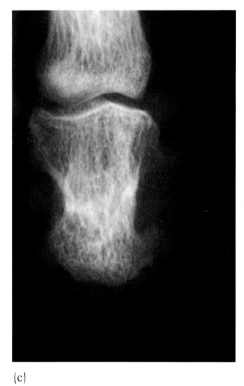

(c)

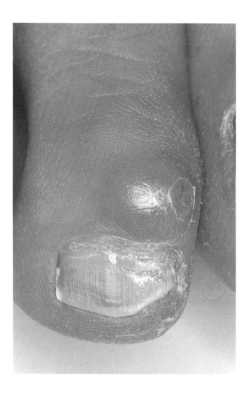

Figure 5.27

Large periungual myxoid pseudocyst.

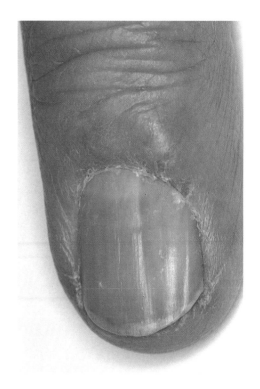

Figure 5.28

Nail plate gutter due to myxoid pseudocyst.

side of the midline and rarely exceed 10–15 mm in diameter. The skin over the lesion is thinned and may be verrucous or even ulcerated. Rarely, paronychial fistula may develop under the proximal nail fold, less commonly under the nail plate. Longitudinal grooving of the nail results from pressure on the matrix. Occasionally a series of irregular transverse grooves are seen, suggesting alternating intermittent decompression and refilling of the cyst. Degenerative, 'wear and tear' osteoarthritis, frequently with Heberden's nodes, is present in most cases.

Histopathology reveals the pseudocystic character. Cavities without synovial lining

> **Myxoid pseudocysts rarely occur without 'wear and tear' osteoarthritis**

are located in an ill defined fibrous capsule. The structure is essentially myxomatous with interspersed fibroblasts. Areas of myxomatous degeneration may merge to form a multilocular pseudocyst. In the cavities, a jelly-like substance is found which stains positively for hyaluronic acid. In some cases a mesothelial-like lining is found in the stalk connecting the pseudocyst with the distal interphalangeal joint. It has been

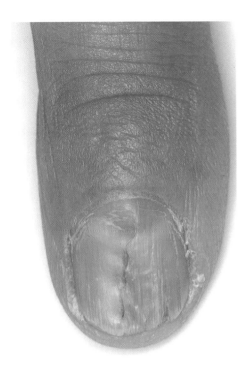

Figure 5.29

Subungual myxoid pseudocyst with nail plate disruption.

suggested that the lesion arises from the joint capsule or tendon sheath synovia, as do ganglia in other areas.

A multitude of treatments have been recommended, including repeated incision and drainage, simple excision, multiple needlings and expression of contents, X-rays (5 Gy, 50 kV, A11 mm, three times at weekly intervals), electrocautery, chemical cautery with nitric acid, trichloroacetic acid or phenol, massages or injection of proteolytic substances, hyaluronidase, steroids (fluoran-drenolone tape, or injections) and sclerosing solutions, cryosurgery, radical excision and even amputation.

The intralesional injection of corticosteroid crystal suspension has been recommended. The cyst is first drained from a proximal point to avoid leakage of the steroid suspension when the patient lowers his hand. Careful dissection and excision of the lesion gives the highest cure rate. A tiny drop of methylene blue solution, diluted with a local anaesthetic and mixed with fresh hydrogen peroxide, is injected into the distal interphalangeal joint at the volar joint crease. The joint will accept only 0.1 to 0.2 ml of dye. This clearly identifies the pedicle connecting the joint to the cyst, if one is present, and also the cyst itself. This procedure sometimes reveals occult satellite cysts. Alternatively the methylene blue may be injected into the cyst to define the tract back to its site of origin. The incision line is drawn on the finger, including a portion of the skin directly over the cyst and continuing proximally in a gentle curve to end dorsally over the joint. The lesion is meticulously dissected from the surrounding soft tissue and the pedicle traced to its origins adjacent to the joint capsule and resected. Dumb-bell extension of cysts to each side of the extensor tendon is easily dissected by hyperextending the joint. Osteophytic spurs adjacent to the joint must be removed with a fine chisel or bone rongeur. Recently, liquid nitrogen cryosurgery has been used with an 86% cure rate. The field treated included the cyst and the adjacent proximal area to the transverse skin creases overlying the terminal joint. Two freeze/thaw cycles were carried out, each freeze time being 30 seconds after the ice field had formed, the intervening thaw time being at least 4 minutes; if this method is adopted then longer freeze times must be avoided or permanent matrix damage may occur. If the cyst is first pricked and emptied of its gelatinous contents, then equally good cure rates can be obtained with a single 20 second freeze after initial ice formation. For distal posterior nail fold lesions, excision of the proximal nail fold and associated cyst has been recommended.

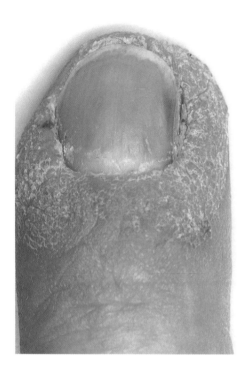

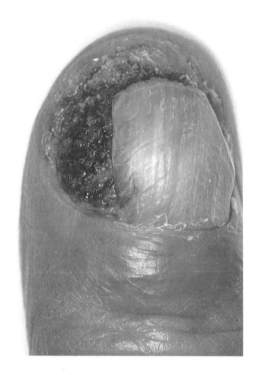

Figure 5.30

Epidermoid carcinoma of the nail apparatus – periungual involvement.

Figure 5.31

Epidermoid carcinoma – subungual involvement.

Sclerosing agents may also be useful: after puncture and expression of cyst contents 0.20–0.30 ml of a 1% solution of sodium tetradecyl sulphate is injected; a second or a third injection may be required at monthly intervals.

Bowen's disease (epidermoid carcinoma)

Bowen's disease is intra-epithelial squamous carcinoma (Figures 5.30–5.32). It is not as rare as might be implied from the medical literature.

> **Intra-epithelial squamous carcinoma is not rare, the whole tumour usually having local invasion at some point.**

The clinical picture of Bowen's disease of the nail unit is variable. It may show a periungual erythematous, squamous or eroded plaque. In the lateral nail wall and groove, it usually presents as a recalcitrant hyperkeratotic or papillomatous, slowly enlarging lesion. Distal involvement of the proximal nail fold results in the formation of a characteristic whitish band.

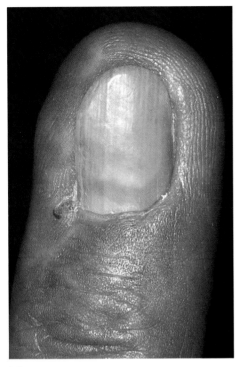

(a)

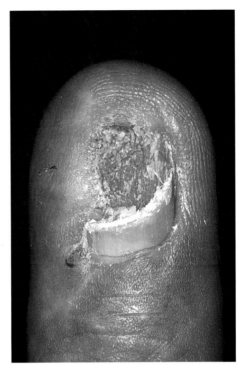

(b)

Figure 5.32

(a) Epidermal carcinoma; (b) epidermal carcinoma – with nail plate trimmed back to show extension of invasion. (Courtesy of G. Cannata.)

The fingers are far more frequently affected than the toes, typically the thumbs, less often the index and middle fingers. The median age at presentation is approximately 60 years, males predominating. Bowen's disease evolves and expands only slowly. Biopsies taken from the most indurated and warty area often reveal invasive squamous cell carcinoma in contrast to the flat plaque. Many authorities therefore no longer differentiate Bowen's disease from squamous cell carcinoma, preferring the term epidermoid carcinoma for all cases.

Surgical removal of the affected area and a small margin of healthy tissue is the treat-ment of choice. With some authorities we prefer the MOHS fresh tissue removal method. Despite the fact that cryosurgery is highly effective in treating Bowen's disease at other skin sites, it is only rarely effective for nail apparatus types.

Squamous cell carcinoma

Squamous cell carcinoma of the nail unit (syn: epidermoid carcinoma) is a low-grade malignancy. Many cases have been reported in the literature, with male predominance.

Trauma, chronic infection and chronic radiation exposure are possible aetiological
factors; HPV virus has been incriminated in
some cases. Two reported cases had associated congenital ectodermal dysplasia. Most
occur on the fingers, particularly the thumbs
and index fingers (Figure 5.31).

> **Squamous cell carcinoma of the nail
> apparatus has a very good prognosis
> compared with other sites**

The presenting symptoms include pain,
swelling, inflammation, elevation of the nail,
ulceration, a tumour 'mass', ingrowing of the
nail, 'pyogenic granuloma' and bleeding.
Bone involvement is a rare, very late sign.
The duration of symptoms before diagnosis
is greater than 12 months in over half the
cases. Only one published case (with ectodermal dysplasia) has led to death, from rapid
generalized metastases.

Subungual squamous cell carcinoma is
slow growing and may be mistaken for
chronic infection. This frequent misdiagnosis unduly prolongs the period between the
onset of the disease, diagnosis and therapy.
Often it is not possible to determine whether
the tumour was present initially or developed later, secondary to trauma, warts or
infection. As mentioned above, invasive
squamous cell carcinoma may develop from
Bowen's disease. The possibility of a link
with HPV 16, 34 and 35 sheds new light on
the aetiology of this type of cancer and
suggests a logical cause for multiple digital
Bowen's disease.

Subungual melanotic lesions

The term longitudinal melanonychia (LM)
describes the presence of single or multiple
longitudinal pigmented streaks within the

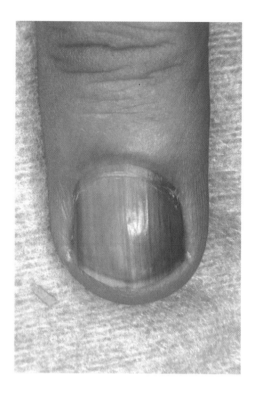

Figure 5.33

Lateral band of LM.

Table 5.5   Causes of longitudinal
melanonychia (LM)

Racial variation
Laugier–Hunziker–Baran syndrome (Figure 5.34)
Inflammatory nail disorders
Drugs
Irradiation
Fungal
Endocrine diseases
Trauma
Neoplasms
AIDS
Nutritional

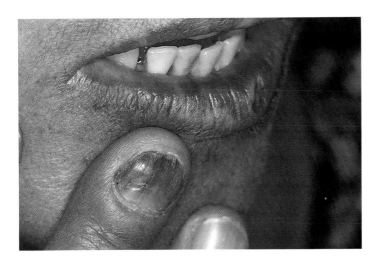

Figure 5.34

Laugier–Hunziker–Baran syndrome –
nail and lip hyperpigmentation.

nail plate (Figure 5.33). A band of LM may
be due to four possible causes:

- Focal activation of the nail matrix
  melanocytes
- Hyperplasia of the nail matrix melano-
  cytes
- Naevus of the nail matrix
- Melanoma of the nail matrix

Table 5.5 lists the causes of LM.

Focal activation of the nail matrix melanocytes

This is the most common cause of LM. In
this variety, the pathology shows
melanocytes with long dendrites located
among nail matrix basal layers. There is no
atypia or theque formation.

Melanocyte activation occurs in 77% of
African-Americans over 20 years of age and
in almost 100% of those over 50. It is
observed in 10 to 20% of Japanese individuals as well as Hispanics and other dark-
skinned groups. It is uncommon in whites.
Variations in racial pigmentation are due to
the number and size of melanosomes
produced. In whites melanosomes are small
and aggregated in complexes. In blacks,
melanosomes are greater in length, larger in
diameter and distributed singly within
keratinocytes.

Melanocyte activation may be induced by
repeated trauma to the nail matrix. Patients
who pick, break or chew the skin over the
proximal nail fold frequently develop bands
of LM. This is usually associated with nail
plate surface abnormalities due to repeated
nail matrix injury. Frictional LM is
commonly observed in the toes of elderly
individuals who have foot deformities and/or
unsatisfactory footwear. The melanonychia
typically appears at the site of friction with
the tip of the shoes or under an overriding
toe (Chapter 9).

Inflammatory disorders of the nail may
also produce nail pigmentation. Post-inflam-
matory melanonychia has been described in
lichen planus, Hallopeau's acrodermatitis
and chronic radiodermatitis. *Trichophyton*

rubrum and *Scytalidium dimidiatum* (Hendersonula toruloidea) nail infection may also occasionally lead to LM. Longitudinal melanonychia may be secondary to the inflammatory changes which induce activation of nail matrix melanocytes, or due to direct melanin production by the fungi.

Activation of nail matrix melanocytes is occasionally seen in endocrine disorders such as Addison's disease, in pregnancy and in patients with HIV infection, even in those not treated with AZT. Nail matrix melanocytes may also be activated by drugs such as AZT, cancer chemotherapeutic agents and psoralens. Drug-induced melanonychia usually involves several digits; it is reversible.

Melanocyte hyperplasia

Melanocyte hyperplasia is characterized by an increased number of melanocytes. Melanocytes are scattered between nail matrix keratinocytes without 'nest' formation. The pathogenesis of melanocyte hyperplasia is unknown. We have found this pathological picture in patients with a single band of LM. Differential diagnosis from melanoma *in situ* may be difficult, and these bands should be completely excised in order to perform serial sections.

Nail matrix naevi

Congenital and acquired melanocytic naevi may occur in the nail matrix and present as LM. Nail matrix naevi are rare and only a few histologically proven naevi of the nail matrix have been reported. Naevi of the nail matrix are most commonly of the junctional type. The architectural pattern of nail matrix naevi is similar to that of skin naevi. Naevus cells are usually seen arranged in nests at the dermo-epidermal junction. Single naevus cells can sometimes be found among nail

matrix basal and suprabasal onychocytes. Dendritic melanocytes are only occasionally present.

HMB-45 staining of nail matrix naevi shows a positive reaction in the cells of the epidermal and junctional component as usually seen in acquired skin naevi. Nail pigmentation due to congenital nail matrix melanocytic naevi may spontaneously regress. However, fading of the pigmentation may only relate to decreased activity of the naevus cells rather than regression of the naevus itself.

The frequency of progression from nail matrix naevi to nail matrix melanoma is not known but a few cases have been well documented. Surgical excision of nail matrix naevi is therefore a justified preventive measure.

Malignant melanoma

In the nail apparatus the most common initial sign of melanoma is acquired LM in white Caucasians or broadening of an existing band in oriental or negroid individuals. This tumour and its practical differential diagnosis from other chromonychias and nail dystrophies is described in this section; linear melanonychia from other causes is considered in Chapter 6.

> **Acquired longitudinal melanonychia after puberty in a white-skinned individual requires urgent biopsy**

Melanoma of the nail region is now better understood since the identification and analysis of acrolentiginous melanoma. It may be localized subungually or periungually with pigmentation and/or dystrophy of the nail plate (Figure 5.35). Initial lesions may be mistaken histologically for benign or atypical melanocytic hyperplasia, but serial sections usually reveal the true nature of the disease.

Approximately 2 to 3% of melanomas in Caucasians, and 15 to 20% in blacks, are located in the nail unit. However, malignant melanoma is rare in Negroes; thus the number of nail melanomas in Caucasians and Negroes does not significantly differ. In Caucasians, most patients have a fair complexion, light hair, and blue or hazel eyes. There is no sex predominance, although some reports show variable female/male predominance. The mean age at onset is 55 to 60 years. Most tumours are found in the thumbs or great toes.

Melanoma of the nail region is often asymptomatic. Many patients only notice a pigmented lesion after trauma to the area; only approximately two-thirds seek medical advice because of the appearance of the lesion; pain or discomfort is rare, and nail deformity, spontaneous ulceration, sudden change in colour, bleeding or tumour mass breaking through the nail are even more infrequent.

It is useful to remember that a pigmented subungual lesion is more likely to be malignant than benign. If the melanoma is pigmented it may show one or more of the following characteristics:

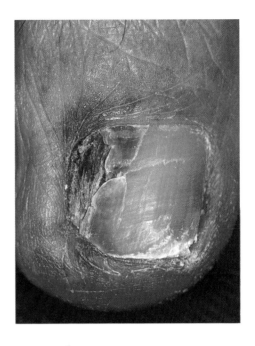

Figure 5.35

Malignant melanoma.

1   A spot, which appears in the matrix, nail bed or plate. This may vary in colour from brown to black: it may be homogeneous or irregular and is seldom painful.
2   A longitudinal brown to black band of variable width running through the whole visible nail.
3   Less frequently, Hutchinson's sign – periungual extension of brown-black pigmentation from LM onto the proximal and lateral nail folds – is an important indicator of subungual melanoma. Current experience, however, has demonstrated that Hutchinson's sign, while valuable, is not an infallible predictor of melanoma, because:

- Periungual pigmentation is present in a variety of benign disorders and, under these circumstances, may lead to overdiagnosis of subungual melanoma.
- Periungual hyperpigmentation occurs in at least one non-melanoma skin cancer: Bowen's disease of the nail unit.
- Hyperpigmentation of the nail bed and matrix may reflect through the 'transparent' nail folds simulating Hutchinson's sign.

'Pseudo-Hutchinson's sign' is a phrase coined to encompass the latter simulant of Hutchinson's sign. Each represents a

Table 5.6 **Disorders accompanied by pseudo-Hutchinson's sign** (after Baran R, Kichijian, P (1996) Hutchinson's sign: a reappraisal, *J Am Acad Dermatol*)

Disorder	Clinical features
Ethnic pigmentation	Proximal nail fold of dark-skinned persons – lateral nail folds not involved. LM may be present or absent. Often exaggerated in thumbs.
Lentigo-naevus	May recur after surgical removal.
Laugier–Hunziker–Baran syndrome	Macular pigmentation of lips, mouth and genitalia. One or several fingers involved.
Peutz–Jegher's syndrome	Hyperpigmentation of fingers and toes, macular pigmentation of buccal mucosa and lips.
X-ray therapy	Treatment for finger dermatitis, psoriasis and chronic paronychia.
Malnutrition	Polydactylus involvement.
Minocycline	Polydactylus involvement.
AIDS patients	Polydactylus involvement. Zidovudine produces similar features.
Trauma-induced	Due to friction, nail biting and picking, boxing.
Bowen's disease	Features clinically typical for subungual melanoma.

misleading clue to the diagnosis of subungual melanoma.

Table 5.6 lists disorders in which pseudo-Hutchinson's sign occurs.

Total reliance on the (apparent) presence or absence of periungual pigmentation may lead to over- or underdiagnosis of subungual melanoma. All relevant clinical and historical information, including the presence or absence of periungual pigmentation, must be carefully evaluated in a patient suspected of having subungual melanoma. Ultimately, the diagnosis of subungual melanoma is made histologically. Hutchinson's sign is a single, important clue to this diagnosis. The nail plate may also become thickened or fissured and permanently shed.

Approximately 25% of melanomas are amelanotic (pigmentation not an obvious or prominent sign, Figures 5.36a,b) and may mimic pyogenic granuloma, granulation

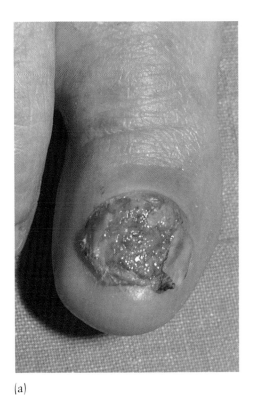

(a)

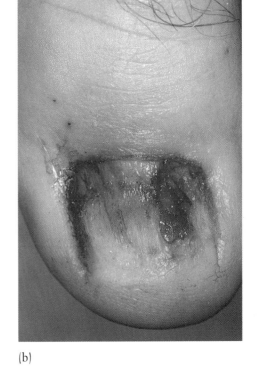

(b)

Figure 5.36

(a,b) Malignant melanoma – amelanotic.

tissue or ingrowing nail. The risk of misdiagnosis is particularly high in these cases.

Malignant melanoma must be considered in the differential diagnosis (see Table 5.3) in all cases of inexplicable chronic paronychia, whether painful or not, in torpid granulomatous ulceration of the proximal nail fold and in pseudoverrucous keratotic lesions of the nail bed and lateral nail groove. Subungual melanoma may also simulate mycobacterial infections, mycotic onychodystrophy, recalcitrant paronychia and ingrowing nail. Subungual haematoma is not rare and may present without a history of severe trauma. It may follow repeated minor trauma which escapes the patient's attention, such as in 'tennis toe', or follow trauma from hard ski boots. Although haematoma following a single traumatic event usually grows out in one piece rather than as a longitudinal streak, due to the continuous production of pigment, repeated trauma may cause difficulties in differential diagnosis. It is recommended that the lesion should be examined with a magnifying loup after it has been covered with a drop of oil. The pigmented nail should be clipped and tested with the argentaffin reaction in order to rule out melanin pigmentation. Subungual haemoglobin is not degraded to haemosiderin and is therefore Prussian blue-negative. Scrapings or small pieces of the nail boiled with water in a test tube give a positive benzidine reaction with the conventional haemostix.

The difference between haemosiderinic and melanotic pigment, sometimes rather difficult to discern by routine histological methods, is easily seen by ultrastructural techniques: ferrous pigment is intercellular while melanin is intracellular.

Because of its frequency, melanonychia striata in deeply pigmented races is considered a normal finding, but up to one-fifth of all melanomas in blacks are in the subungual area, and these typically begin with a pigmented spot producing a longitudinal streak. These spots are usually black rather than the normal brown. The diagnosis may be aided by comparing them with the brown stripes in other nails or by the occurrence of Hutchinson's sign.

The following guidelines should be adhered to where possible to enable accurate tissue diagnosis to be made and appropriate treatment carried out.

As a first step, the anatomical site of the matrix affected will be obtained from the level of the melanin pigment identified with Fontana's silver stain of a nail clipping obtained from the distal free edge. The type of biopsy selected will then depend on:

• The site of the matrix melanin production.
• The width of the linear pigmentation.
• The site of the band in the nail plate.

If the pigment is located within the ventral portion of the nail plate, a decision has to be made depending on the width of the band:

• A punch biopsy should be used when the width of the band is less than 3 mm. If the base of the nail plate is removed, the specimen may be released more easily, and the integrity of the region distal to the biopsied matrix area may be checked.
• A transverse matrix biopsy should be used for a band wider than 3 mm.

If the pigment involves the upper portion of the nail, it is obviously difficult to use the two previous procedures to remove the source of melanin pigment, for anatomical reasons and because of the risk of a secondary dystrophy, thus:

• A rectangular block of tissue is excised using two parallel incisions down to the bone. An L-shaped incision is carried back along the lateral nail wall, freeing this flap. The lateral section may then be rotated medially and approximated to the remaining nail segment.
• If the band is wider than 6 mm or if the whole thickness of the nail is involved by the pigment, surgical removal of the nail apparatus seems the most logical method. However, one (or even two) 3 mm punch biopsy is an alternative prior to more radical treatment, especially in young women.
• When the band lies within the lateral third of the nail plate, lateral longitudinal biopsy is more suitable.
• If LM is accompanied by periungual pigmentation (Hutchinson's sign), removal of the nail apparatus is required.

Histological examination of acral lentiginous melanoma requires great experience, and often serial sections are needed to classify the lesion accurately. Grading according to Clark's levels or Breslow's maximum tumour thickness is difficult and often inconclusive.

> **Nail apparatus melanoma has a poor prognosis, with up to 50% of patients dying within 5 years of the diagnosis**

Subungual melanoma has a poor prognosis. The reported 5-year survival rates are from 35 to 50%. Most patients present with advanced subungual melanoma; however,

Table 5.7   **Conditions in which nail pustulation may occur**

Infective (primary cause)	Acute paronychia (see page 89) Blistering distal dactylitis Hand–foot–mouth disease Herpes simplex (primary and recurrent) Gonorrhoea Impetigo *Veillonella* infection – newborn

Non-infective (secondary infection may occur)	Ingrowing toe nail
	    Malalignment in childhood
	    Common type
	Self-inflicted bullous lesions of newborn
	Thumb sucking (and paronychia)

Dermatoses	Acrokeratosis paraneoplastica Acropustulosis/psoriasis Parakeratosis pustulosa Reiter's syndrome

even early diagnosis is not a guarantee of a good prognosis. Women have a better prognosis than men.

Factors which contribute to a poor prognosis are delay in diagnosis and, as a result of this, inadequate treatment. The tumour may be mistaken for a traumatic dystrophy, and valuable time may be lost before the diagnosis is made. Treatment depends on the stage of the disease. Levels I and II melanomas may be adequately treated by wide local excision, and repair of the defect with graft or flap. Amputation is usually advised for melanoma at levels more advanced than II. When the thumb is affected and therefore amputated, pollicization of a finger may provide a functional replacement. There would appear to be no relationship between the prognosis and the extent of the amputation, although metacarpo/metatarsophalangeal amputation is considered to be inadequate because of local recurrences. The rationale for elective lymph node dissection and/or isolated hyperthermic perfusion of the extremity with cytotoxic drugs is still under discussion. Immune enhancement such as BCG therapy is used in some centres.

Pustules

The conditions in which nail apparatus pustulation may be a significant sign are listed in Table 5.7.

Herpes simplex

Distal digital herpes simplex infection may affect the terminal phalanx as a primary

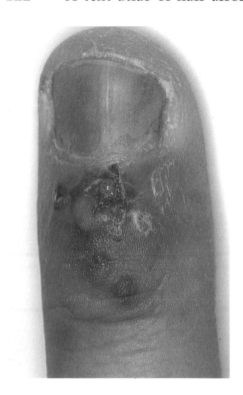

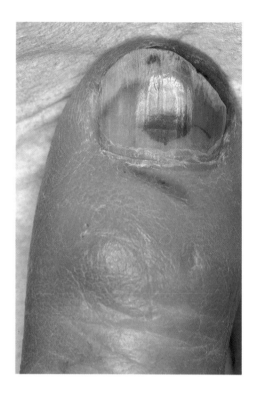

Figure 5.37

Primary herpes simplex – herpetic 'whitlow'.

Figure 5.38

Subungual recurrent herpes simplex.

herpetic 'whitlow' or start as an acute, intensely painful, paronychia (Figures 5.37, 5.38). It is relatively common in dental staff, anaesthetists and those involved with the care of the mouth and upper respiratory tract in unconscious patients. Recurrent forms are generally less severe and have a milder clinical course than the initial infection.

After an incubation period of 3 to 7 days, during which local tenderness, erythema and swelling may develop, a crop of vesicles appears at the site of origin in the skin. The vesicles are typically distributed in the paronychia and on the volar digital skin, resembling pyogenic infection of the fingertip. Close inspection, however, will reveal the classic pale, raised vesicles surrounded by an erythematous border. An acutely painful 'whitlow' may develop and extend under the distal free edge of the nail and into the nail bed. A distinct predilection for the thumb, index and ring fingers on the dominant hand has been noted, but any finger may be involved. Multiple lesions are rare. For 10 to 14 days the vesicles gradually increase in size, often coalescing into large, honeycombed bullae. New crops of lesions may appear during this time. Vesicular fluid is clear early in the disease but may become turbid, seropurulent or even haemorrhagic within days of onset. At times, a pale yellow colour of the vesicles will suggest pyogenic infection, yet frank pus is not usually obtained. Patients complain of tenderness and severe throbbing in the affected digit. Coexisting primary herpetic infections of the mouth and fingernails suggest auto-inoculation of the virus into the nail tissues as a result of nail biting or finger sucking.

Radiating pain along the C7 distribution is sometimes noted before each recurrence. Lymphangitis may start from the wrist and extend to the axilla with painful lymphadenopathy. Numbness and hypuaesthesia following the acute episode have been observed.

The diagnosis of herpetic infection can be made by examining the base of the vesicles for the characteristic multinucleated 'balloon' giant cells, in stained smears. The presence of intranuclear inclusions is also significant. Viral cultivation, usually positive within 24 hours of onset, is confirmatory; the active viral phase lasts up to 4 to 5 days in primary attacks but only 2 to 3 days in recurrent episodes.

Differential diagnosis

It is important to exclude primary or recurrent herpes simplex infection in the differential diagnosis of every vesiculopustular finger infection. The typical appearance of the lesions with disproportionately severe pain, the absence of pus in the confluent, multiloculated, vesiculopustular lesions and the lack of increased tension in the finger pulp aid in differentiating this slow healing infection from a bacterial foreign body or paronychia.

Herpes zoster infections, which may affect the proximal nail fold like herpes simplex, also involve the entire sensory dermatome. The pustules of primary cutaneous *Neisseria* *gonorrhoeae* infection may resemble herpes simplex on the rare occasion when it occurs on the finger. The diagnosis is established by positive Gram stain and bacteriological culture.

Treatment is aimed primarily at symptomatic relief and the avoidance of secondary infection. Topical acyclovir may shorten the course of any one attack; given orally the drug may prevent recurrences whilst it is being taken. On cessation of the treatment relapses are unfortunately common. This is a preventable infection. Gloves should always be worn on both hands for procedures such as intubation, removal of dentures or providing oral care, despite the additional costs involved.

Subungual infection in the newborn due to Veillonella

Many epidemics of subungual infection have been described among infants in postnatal wards and special care baby units. The number of fingers affected per patient ranged from one to ten; the thumbs are less frequently involved than other fingers; toe nails are not affected. Three stages occur: first, a small amount of clear fluid appears under the centre of the nail, along with mild inflammation at the distal end of the finger. This initial vesicle lasts approximately 24 hours; it sometimes enlarges but never to the edge of the nail. Some small lesions bypass the second, pustular stage, going directly to the third stage. As a rule the fluid becomes yellow after 24 hours, the pus remaining for 24 to 48 hours, before gradually turning brown, and being absorbed. This colour fades progressively over a period of 2 to 6 weeks, leaving the nail and nail bed completely normal.

Subungual pus obtained by aseptic puncture of the nails showed tiny, gram-negative cocci about 0.4 µm in diameter.

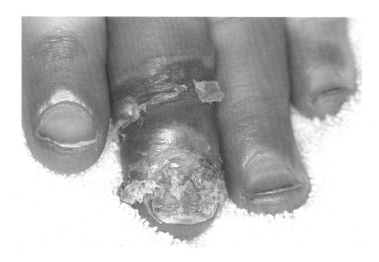

Figure 5.39

Impetigo of the nail apparatus.

These organisms resemble *Veillonella*, a group of anaerobes of dubious pathogenicity found as commensals in the saliva, vagina and respiratory tract. Systemic antibiotics do not change the clinical course of the nail lesions, which do not differ from those observed in other untreated and affected newborn children.

Impetigo

The dorsal aspect of the distal phalanx may be involved by impetigo (Figure 5.39). It presents in two forms:

1 Vesiculopustular, with its familiar honey-crusted lesions, usually due to β-haemolytic streptococci
2 Bullous, usually due to phage type 71 staphylococci

The latter is characterized by the appearance of large, localized, intraepidermal bullae that persist for longer periods than the transient vesicles of streptococcal impetigo which subsequently rupture spontaneously to form very thin crusts.

The lesions of bullous impetigo may mimic the non-infectious bullous diseases (such as drug-induced types or pemphigoid). Oral therapy of bullous impetigo with a penicillinase-resistant penicillin should be instituted and continued until the lesions resolve. Cephalexin and erythromycin are acceptable alternatives. The lesions should be cleansed several times daily and topical aureomycin (3%) applied to all the affected areas.

Blistering distal dactylitis

Blistering distal dactylitis (BDD) is a variant of streptococcal skin infection. It presents as a superficial, tender, blistering β-haemolytic streptococcal infection over the anterior fat pad of the distal phalanx of the finger (Figure 5.40). The lesion may or may not have a

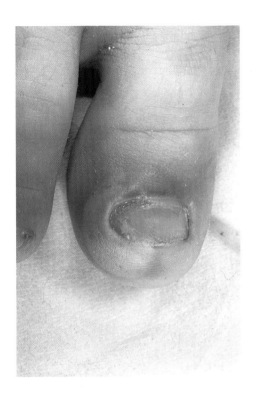

Figure 5.40

Blistering distal dactylitis.

paronychial extension. This blister, containing thin, white pus, has a predilection for the tip of the digit and extends to the subungual area of the free edge of the nail plate. The area may provide a nidus for the β-haemolytic streptococcus and act as a focus of chronic infection similar to the nasopharynx. The age range of affected patients is 2 to 16 years. For local care incision, drainage and antiseptic soaking are indicated, giving a more rapid response than systemic antibiotic therapy alone: effective regimes include benzathine penicillin G in a single intramuscular dose, a 10-day course of oral phenoxymethyl penicillin or erythromycin ethyl succinate. This type of treatment decreases the reservoir of streptococci by preventing spread to family contacts. This infection has been described as a complication of ingrowing toe nail.

The differential diagnosis includes blisters resulting from friction, thermal and chemical burns, infectious states such as herpetic whitlow, staphylococcal bullous impetigo and the Weber-Cokayne variant of epidermolysis bullosa simplex.

Chronic paronychia and thumb sucking

Candida paronychia, usually in association with oral candidosis, may arise as a result of chronic maceration due to thumb sucking (Figure 5.41). Chronic paronychia is not uncommon in children. It differs from the condition seen in adults in the source of the maceration, associated diseases, the clinical appearances of the lesion, and the patient's responses to the symptoms. In children the lesions are generally very prominent, with total involvement of the proximal nail fold. The skin is usually erythematous and glistening due to the wet environment produced by continuous thumb sucking. The quality of the nail is always altered, resulting in a poor texture. The habit of sucking fingers or thumbs is the most important predisposing factor. *Candida albicans* is present in all cases. When an acute flare-up occurs the patient experiences pruritus and discomfort in the proximal nail fold. Children respond to this by sucking – the symptoms of chronic paronychia perpetuating the habit which intiated the maceration. The lesions tend to be more severe in childhood than in adult paronychia, probably because thumb sucking is more continuous than exposure to wet work, and saliva is

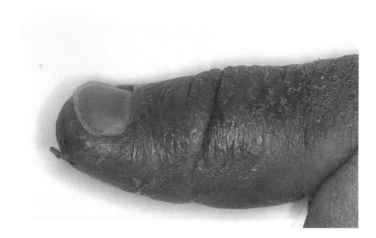

Figure 5.41

Chronic paronychia and thumb
sucking – atopic individual.

more irritating than water. The minor
repeated trauma resulting from suction is
capable of causing complete loss of the nail
plate. Detection of the carrier state in the
mouth and gastrointestinal tract by cultures
of saliva and stools may be important in the
occasional patient with refractory paronychia. Persistent and repeated candida paronychia in infancy suggests a more serious
underlying disorder and such infants should
be investigated for endocrine disease and
immune deficiency syndromes.

Thumb or finger sucking is sometimes
associated with herpes simplex. This may
result in local extension of the eruption
producing viral stomatitis combined with
involvement of the digit. In childhood, local
trauma, caused by onychophagia, may result
in the development of opportunistic infection by the normal oropharyngeal flora,
amongst which are found HB 1 bacteria.
Acute paronychia may also be caused by HB
1 organisms (*Eikenella corrodens*), but this is
uncommon in the absence of immune
deficiency.

Acropustuloses/pustular psoriasis

In pustular psoriasis and acrodermatitis
continua (Hallopeau's disease), involvement
of a single digit is common. It is often misdi-
agnosed when the pustule appears beneath
the nail plate with necrosis of tissue resulting in desiccation and crust formation. New
pustule formation may develop at the periph-
ery or within the lesions. The nail is lifted
off by the crust and lakes of pus and new
pustules may form on the denuded nail bed
(Figures 5.42–5.44). Permanent loss is possible. Acral pustular psoriasis has been
reported with resorptive osteolysis ('deep
Koebner phenomenon') and pronounced skin
and subcutaneous tissue atrophy. There may
be progressive loss of entire digits in the feet
and loss of fingertips and finger nails. 'Tuft'
osteolysis may occur independently of
acropustuloses and arthritis. Histopathology
reveals Munro-Sabouraud 'micro-abscesses'
or the spongiform pustule of Kogoj.

Localized PUVA can be of benefit. Oral
retinoid therapy may give good short-term

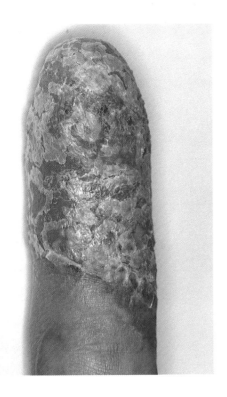

Figure 5.42

Psoriatic acropustulosis (Hallopeau).

results, but recurrences appear 1 to 3 months after the treatment has been stopped. Combined retinoid and PUVA treatment delays and lowers the frequency of relapses. Topical mechloretamine has given some good results as has intramuscular triamcinolone acetonide.

The differential diagnosis of acropustulosis may be controversial, particularly with regard to the subcorneal pustular dermatosis of Sneddon and Wilkinson. Many authorities have described patients with pustular lesions like those described as subcorneal pustular dermatosis, but who had in addition stigmata suggestive of psoriasis. These included typical scaly plaques on the elbows and knees, pitted nails or arthropathy. It is, however, pointless to debate the pathogenesis of Sneddon–Wilkinson disease without applying the techniques available for identifying the psoriatic state: cell kinetics, complement activation in the stratum corneum, HLA family studies and nail growth studies.

Figure 5.43

Pustular psoriasis.

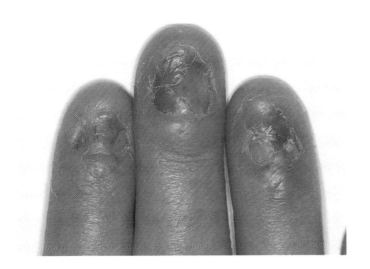

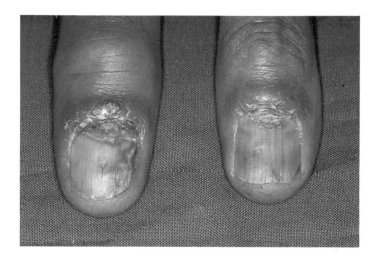

Figure 5.44

Proximal pustular psoriasis – limited form of acropustulosis.

Reiter's syndrome

> **All the nail signs in Reiter's syndrome may be present in severe psoriasis**

The clinical and histological features of the skin changes in Reiter's syndrome may be indistinguishable from those of psoriasis. Skin changes resembling paronychia can accompany nail involvement, suggesting inflammation of the proximal nail fold. Onycholysis, ridging, splitting, greenish-yellow or sometimes brownish-red discoloration and subungual hyperkeratosis may be present. Small yellow pustules may develop and slowly enlarge beneath the nail, often near the lunula. Their contents become dry and brown. The nails may be shed. Nail pitting may be seen in Reiter's syndrome, individual pits being deep and punched out. This nail pitting may reflect a predisposition to the development of psoriasis or psoriasiform lesions dependent on the HLA-A2 and B 27 antigens, as suggested by previously reported HLA typing studies. HLA-A2 and B 27 were present in a 6-year-old boy who had only the nail changes which were compatible with Reiter's syndrome; the same antigens were also present in his father, who had uveitis, arthritis and amyloidosis.

Antibiotics, steroids and non-steroidal anti-inflammatory drugs are without benefit. PUVA may be helpful. Oral retinoid therapy may clear the nails in Reiter's syndrome. Combined chemotherapy with methotrexate, oral retinoid and prednisolone has been suggested.

Parakeratosis pustulosa (Hjorth–Sabouraud syndrome)

This parakeratotic condition of the fingertip was first described more than 50 years ago. It usually occurs in girls of approximately 7 years of age, typically affecting only one digit, usually a finger (Figure 5.45). The lesions start close to the free margin of the nail of a

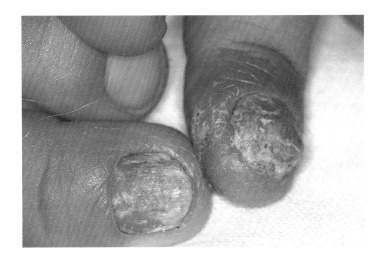

Figure 5.45

Parakeratosis pustulosa.

finger or toe. In some cases, a few isolated pustules or vesicles may be observed in the initial phase; these usually disappear before the patient presents to the doctor. Confluent eczematoid changes cover the skin immediately adjacent to the distal edge of the nail. The affected area is pink or of normal skin colour and densely studded with fine scales; there is a clear margin between the normal and affected areas. The skin changes may extend to the dorsal aspect of the finger or toe, but usually only the fingertip is affected. The most striking and characteristic change is the hyperkeratosis beneath the nail tip. The nail plate is lifted up, deformed and often thickened. Commonly the deformity produced is asymmetrical and limited to one corner of the distal edge, or at least more pronounced at the corners of the nail. Pitting occurs in some cases; rarely transverse ridging of the nail plate is present. Most cases resolve within a few months, but some cases persist for many years, even into adult life.

Histological findings are of some value, including hyperkeratosis and parakeratosis, pustulation and crusts, acanthosis and mild exocytosis, papillomatosis and heavy cellular infiltrates composed mainly of lymphocytes and fibroblasts around dilated capillary loops. This histology presents many of the features common to psoriasis and eczema.

In the differential diagnosis of parakeratosis pustulosa, the following points are important:

- Pustules are very rare and only seen in the initial stage, as distinct from pustular psoriasis or acropustulosis.
- Patients with psoriasis develop a coarse sheet of scales and not the fine type of scaling typically seen in parakeratosis pustolosa.
- If the nail changes predominate, especially on a toe, the disorder can be mistaken for onychomycosis. Thumb sucking, which is a predisposing factor in chronic candidal paronychia, should be ruled out when a single thumb is affected.

No treatment makes any difference to the frequency of recurrence or the overall

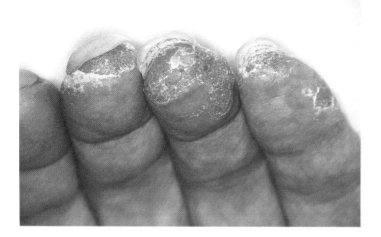

Figure 5.46

Acrokeratosis paraneoplastica.

duration of parakeratosis pustulosa. Topical steroids provide some symptomatic relief.

Acrokeratosis paraneoplastica of Bazex and Dupré

Acrokeratosis paraneoplastica occurs in association with malignant epithelial tumours of the upper respiratory or digestive tracts, in particular the pharyngolaryngeal area pyriform fossa, tonsillar area, epiglottis, hard and soft palate, vocal cords, tongue, lower lip, oesophagus and the upper third of the lungs. It also occurs with metastases to the cervical and upper mediastinal lymph nodes. This 'paraneoplasia' may precede the signs of the associated malignancy, disappear when the tumour is removed and reappear with its recurrence; however, the nail involvement does not always benefit from total recovery, in contrast to the other lesions. This condition almost exclusively occurs in men over 40 years of age. The lesions are erythematous, violaceous and keratotic with ill defined borders. They are symmetrically distributed, affecting hands, feet, ears and occasionally the nose. The toe nails suffer more severely than the finger nails. Roughened, irregular, keratotic, fissured and warty excrescences are found equally on the terminal phalanges of both fingers and toes (Figure 5.46).

The nails are invariably involved and are typically the earliest manifestation of the disease. In mild forms, the nail involvement is discrete; the affected nails are thin, soft and may become fragile and crumble. In more established disease, the nails are flaky, irregular, whitened and the free edge is raised by subungual hyperkeratosis. In severe forms, the lesions resemble advanced psoriatic nail dystrophy and may progress to complete loss of the diseased nails. The nail bed is eventually replaced by a smooth epidermis to which the irregular, horny vestiges of the nail still adhere. The periungual skin shows an erythemato-squamous eruption, predominantly on the dorsum of the terminal phalanges; there may be associated chronic paronychia with occasional, acute suppurative exacerbations.

The two extremes of the disease may coexist. In these cases, the proximal third of the nail is atrophic and the distal two-thirds exhibits hypertrophic changes. The histopathological changes are non-specific, though they do enable the exclusion of a diagnosis of psoriasis, lupus erythematosus or other similar eruptions.

Miscellaneous dermatoses

Virtually all skin diseases can sometimes affect the paronychial tissue. It is therefore wise to examine the entire skin of a patient presenting with lesions of the perungual skin.

Further reading

Paronychia

Baran R, Bureau H (1983) Congenital malalignment of the big toe-nail as a cause of ingrowing toe-nail in infancy. Pathology and treatment (a study of thirty cases), *Clin Exp Dermatol* **8**: 619–623.

Barth JH, Dawber RPR (1987) Diseases of the nails in children, *Pediatr Dermatol* **4**: 275–290.

Editorial (1975) Chronic paronychia, *BMJ* **ii**: 460.

Stone OJ, Mullins JF, Head ES (1964) Chronic paronychia. Occupational material, *Arch Environ Health* **9**: 585–588.

Stone OJ, Mullins FJ (1968) Chronic paronychia in children, *Clin Pediatr* **7**: 104–107.

Tosti A, Guerra L, Morelli R, Bardazzi F, Fanti PA (1992) Role of foods in the pathogenesis of chronic paronychia, *J Am Acad Dermatol* **27**: 706–710.

Zaias N (1990) *The Nail in Health and Disease*, 2nd edn (Appleton and Lange: East Norwalk).

Tumours and swellings

Baran R, Kichijian P (1989) Longitudinal melanonychia. Diagnosis and management. *J Am Acad Dermatol* **21**: 1165–1175.

Baran R, Kichijian P (1996) Hutchinson's sign: a reappraisal. *J Am Acad Dermatol* (in press).

Briggs JC (1985) Subungual malignant melanoma: a review article, *Br J Plast Surg* **38**: 174–176.

Salasche SJ, Garland LD (1985) Tumours of the nail, *Dermatol Clin* **3**: 501–519.

Pustules

Hjorth N, Thomsen K (1967) Parakeratosis pustulosa, *Br J Dermatol* **79**: 527–532.

6 Nail consistency

Fragile, brittle and soft nails

Many of the nail diseases which disrupt nail formation and structure cause 'secondary' brittleness and fragility. In this chapter only those conditions leading to nail fragility or brittleness as a major sign are considered in any detail (Figures 6.1–6.7).

'Hapalonychia' is the term used for crypto-genic soft nail – those cases for which there is no primary specific local nail disease to explain the change. Diseases and conditions associated with this include:

- Congenital types
- Sulphur deficiency syndromes
- Thin nail plate of any cause
- Occupational disease (for example working with industrial oils)
- Chronic arthritis
- Leprosy
- Hypothyroidism
- Peripheral ischaemia
- Peripheral neuritis
- Hemiplegia
- Cachexic states.

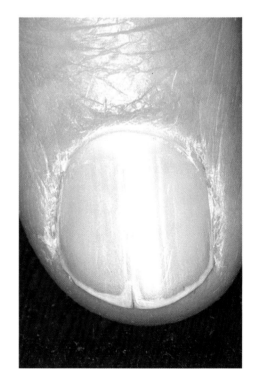

Figure 6.1

Distal nail fissure.

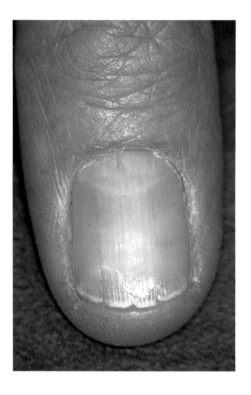

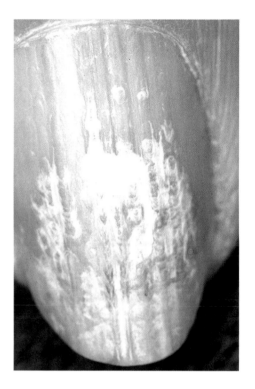

Figure 6.2

Distal nail fragility.

Figure 6.3

Surface nail fragility and fractures due to nail varnish (keratin granulations).

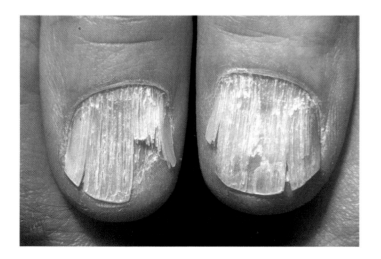

Figure 6.4

Nail fragility in lichen planus.

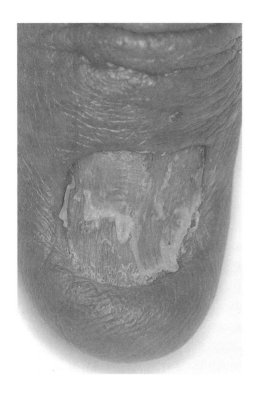

Figure 6.5

Severe nail plate fragility and loss.

In some cases of hapalonychia the thinned nails assumed a semi-transparent, bluish-white hue, sometimes described as 'egg-shell nails'.

Brittle nails can be divided into four main types on morphological grounds:

1 An isolated split at the free edge which sometimes extends proximally. This may result from onychorrhexis with shallow parallel furrows running in the superficial layer of the nail.
2 Multiple, crenellated splitting which resembles the battlements of a castle. Triangular pieces may easily be torn from the free margin.
3 Lamellar splitting of the free edge of the nail into fine layers (*see* Figures 3.25, 3.27). This may occur alone or associated with the other types.
4 Transverse splitting and breaking of the lateral edge close to the distal margin.

The changes in brittle, friable nails are often confined to the surface of the nail plate; this occurs in superficial white onychomycosis and may be seen after the

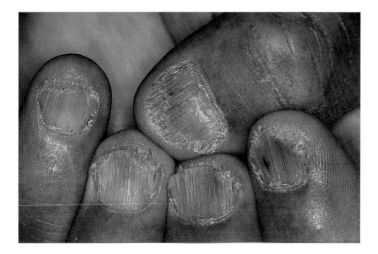

Figure 6.6

Nail apparatus – amyloidosis.

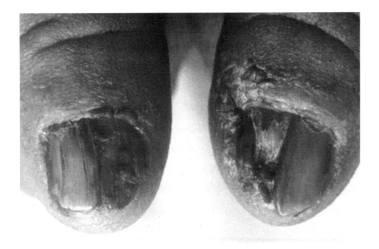

Figure 6.7

Darier's disease with some nail plate loss.

application of nail polish or base coat which causes 'granulations' in the nail keratin. In advanced psoriasis and fungal infection the friability may extend throughout the entire nail.

The changes in nail consistency may be due to impairment of one or more of the factors on which the health of the nail depends, for example variations in the water content or keratin structures. In addition, changes in the intercellular structures and cell membranes, and intracellular changes in the arrangement of keratin fibrils have been revealed by electron microscopy. Normal nails contain approximately 18% water. After prolonged immersion in water this percentage is increased and the nail becomes soft; this makes toe nail trimming and nail biopsies much easier. A low lipid content may decrease the nail's ability to retain water. If the water content is considerably reduced, the nail becomes brittle. Splitting, which results from this brittle quality, is probably partly due to repeated uptake and loss of water.

The keratin content may be modified by chemical and physical insults, especially in occupational nail disorders. Amino acid chains may be broken or distorted by alkalis, oxidizing agents and thioglycolates, as employed in the permanent waving processes. These break or distort the multiple-S–S-bond linkages which join the protein chains to form the keratin fibrils. Keratin structure can also be changed in genetic disorders, such as dyskeratosis congenita in which the nail plate is completely absent, or reduced to thin, dystrophic remnants.

The composition of the nail plate is sometimes related to generalized disease. High sulphur content in the form of cystine predominates, which contributes to the stability of the fibrous protein by the formation of disulphide bonds. A lack of iron can result in softening of the nail and koilonychia; conversely, the calcium content in the nail would appear to contribute little towards its hardness. Calcium is located mainly in the surface of the nail, in small absorbed quantities, and X-ray diffraction shows no evidence of calcite or apatite crystals.

Damage to both the central and peripheral nervous system may result in nail fragility.

Table 6.1 Factors leading to fragile, brittle or soft nails

Local factors
 Trauma
  Occupational
  Onychotillomania
 Chemical

Dermatological conditions which may thin the nail plate
 Alopecia areata
 Amyloidosis
 Darier's disease
 Eczema
 Lichen planus
 Lichen striatus
 Onychomycosis
 Psoriasis
 Slow nail growth

General factors
 Anaemia (iron deficiency)
 Cachexic state
 Chronic arthropathies (fingers or toes)
 Drugs
  Antimetabolites
  Arsenic
  Acitretine-etretinate
  Gold salts
  Peloprenoic acid
  Penicillamine
  Vitamin A, C and B_6 deficiencies
 Gout
 Graft versus host disease
 Haemodialysis
 Hyper- or hypothyroidism
 Neurological
  Hemiplegia
  Neuropathies
 Osteomalacia
 Osteoporosis
 Peripheral circulatory impairment (arterial)
 Pregnancy
 Sulphur deficiency diseases

Local causes

The nail may be damaged by trauma or by chemical agents such as detergents, alkalis, various solvents, sugar solutions and especially by hot water.

The nail plate takes a minimum of 5 to 6 months to regenerate and therefore it is vulnerable to daily insults. The housewife is very susceptible; particularly at risk are the first three fingers of the dominant hand. Anything which slows the rate of nail growth will increase the risk. Cosmetic causes are rare. Some varnishes will damage the superficial layers of the nail. Drying may be enhanced by some nail varnish removers and soaking fingers in warm soapy solution, for removing the cuticle, is especially dangerous; this is common practice among manicurists. It has been shown that climatic and seasonal factors may affect the hydration of the nail plate.

Fragility, due to thinning of the nail plate, may be caused by a reduction in the length of the matrix. Diminution, or even complete arrest of nail formation over a variable width may be the result of many dermatoses such as eczema, lichen planus, psoriasis (rare) and impairment of the peripheral circulation. The frequency of nail fragility in alopecia areata lends credence to the popular belief that nail and hair disorders are often associated.

General causes

These are listed in Table 6.1. The diverse constituents of the nail plate, especially the enzymes necessary for the formation of keratin, are subject to genetic influences; changes in these are exhibited in the form of hereditary disease.

7 Nail colour changes (chromonychia)

The term 'chromonychia' indicates an abnormality in colour of the substance, or the surface of the nail plate and/or subungual tissues. Generally, abnormalities of colour depend on the transparency of the nail, its attachments and the character of the underlying tissues. Pigment may accumulate due to overproduction (melanin) or storage (haemosiderin, copper, various drugs), or by surface deposition. The nails provide a historical record for up to 2 years (depending on the rate of linear nail growth) of profound temporary abnormalities of the control of skin pigment which otherwise might pass unnoticed. Colour is also affected by the state of the skin vessels, and various intravascular factors such as anaemia and carbon monoxide poisoning.

> **Complex internal diseases may sometimes be diagnosed solely by colour changes in the nail apparatus**

There are some important points to note concerning the examination of abnormal nails for colour changes. They should be studied with the fingers completely relaxed and not pressed against any surface. Failure to do this alters the haemodynamics of the nail and changes its appearance. The fingertip should then be blanched to see if the pigmented abnormality is grossly altered; this may help to differentiate between discoloration of the nail plate and its vascular bed. If the discoloration is in the vascular bed, it will usually disappear. Further information can be gleaned by transillumination of the nail using a pen torch placed against the pulp. If the discoloration is in the matrix or soft tissue, the exact position can be identified more easily. Furthermore, if a topical agent is suspected as the cause, one can remove the discoloration by scraping or cleaning the nail plate with a solvent such as acetone. If the substance is impregnated more deeply into the nail or subungually, microscopic studies of potassium hydroxide preparations or biopsy specimens using special stains may be indicated. Wood's lamp examination is sometimes useful.

When there is nail contact with occupationally derived agents, or topical application of therapeutic agents, the discoloration typically follows the contour of the proximal nail fold. If the discoloration corresponds to the shape of the lunula an internal cause is likely.

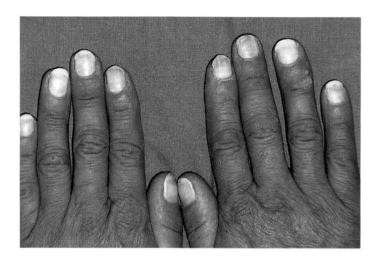

Figure 7.1

Leukonychia – hereditary type.

Leukonychia (white nail)

White nails are the most common colour change seen. These can be divided into two main types:

1 True leukonychia, in which the nail plate is involved
2 Apparent leukonychia with involvement of the subungual tissue.

In true leukonychia (Figure 7.1) the nail appears opaque and white in colour owing to the diffraction of light in the abnormal keratotic cells; with polarized light, the nail structure appears disrupted due to disorganization of the keratin fibrils. The leukonychia may be complete, total leukonychia (rare), or incomplete, subtotal leukonychia. These forms can be temporary or permanent depending on the aetiology. Partial forms are divided into punctate leukonychia, which is common, striate leukonychia, relatively common, and distal leukonychia, which is very rare. The term 'pseudoleukonychia' is used when fungal infection involves the nail plate, for example in superficial white onychomycoses, or when nail varnish produces keratin granulation. Apparent leukonychia can be further subdivided into a white appearance of the nail due to:

1 Underlying onycholysis and subungual hyperkeratosis
2 Modification of the matrix and/or the nail bed, giving rise, for example, to apparent macrolunula.

True leukonychia

Total leukonychia

In this rare condition (Figure 7.1) the nail may be milky, chalky, bluish, ivory or porcelain white in colour. The opacity of the whiteness varies: when it is faintly opaque, it may be possible to see transverse streaks of leukonychia in a nail with total leukonychia. A transition to black has been observed

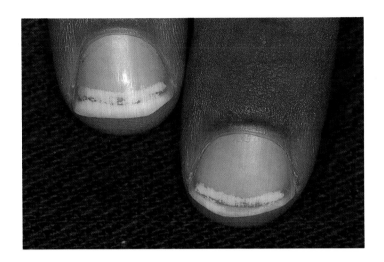

Figure 7.2

Leukonychia – transverse banded type.

in the distal nail plate portion in patients suffering from severe cholestatic jaundice. Accelerated nail growth may be associated with total leukonychia.

Subtotal leukonychia

In this form, there is a pink arc of about 2–4 mm width distal to the white area. This can be explained by the fact that the nucleated cells in the distal area mature, lose their keratohyalin granules and then produce healthy keratin several weeks after their formation. It is possible that parakeratotic cells are present along the whole length of the nail; these decrease in number as they approach the distal end, thus producing the normal pink colour up to the point of separation from the nail bed. There might, however, be sufficient remaining for the nail to acquire a whitish tint after loss of contact with the nail bed. Some authorities feel that subtotal leukonychia is a phase of total leukonychia based on the occurrence of both types in different members of one family and

the simultaneous occurrence in one person. In addition, either type may be found alone in some individuals at different times.

Transverse leukonychia

One or several nails exhibit a band, usually transverse, 1–2 mm wide and often occurring at the same site in each nail (Figure 7.2, 7.3). Transverse leukonychia is almost always due to trauma affecting the distal matrix (for example) due to overzealous manicuring.

Multiple transverse leukonychia may involve the great toes or the second toe nails. In these patients whose nails are never trimmed short, the free margin is presumed to impinge on the distal part of the shoe. Cutting the affected nails short leads to complete cure.

Punctate leukonychia

In this type, white spots of 1–3 mm in diameter occur singly or in groups; only

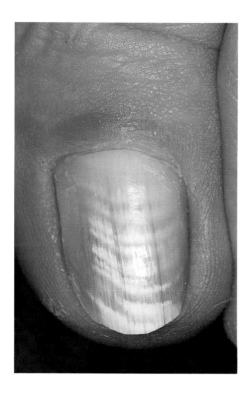

Figure 7.3

Extensive variant of the type in Figure 7.2.

rarely do they occur on toe nails. They are usually due to repeated, minor trauma to the matrix. The evolution of the spots is variable; appearing generally on contact with the cuticle, they grow distally with the nail but approximately 50% disappear as they migrate towards the free edge. This proves that parakeratotic cells are capable of maturing and losing their keratohyalin granules to produce keratin, even though they have been without a blood supply for many months. Some white spots enlarge whilst others appear at a distance from the lunula, suggesting that the nail bed is participating by incorporating groups of nucleated cells into the

nail. A similar process could explain the exclusively distal leukonychia which is occasionally seen. A local or general fault in keratinization is not the only cause of punctate leukonychia; infiltration of air, which is known to occur in cutaneous parakeratoses, may also play a part.

Leukonychia variegata

This consists of white, irregular, transverse, thread-like streaks.

Isolated longitudinal leukonychia

Isolated longitudinal leukonychia is an example of localized metaplasia. It is characterized by a permanent greyish white longitudinal streak, 1 mm broad, below the nail plate. Histologically there is a mound of horny cells causing the white discoloration due to a lack of transparency leading to alteration in light diffraction.

Apparent leukonychia

White opacity of the nails in patients with cirrhosis is often known as Terry's nail. In the majority of cases, the nails are of an opaque white colour, obscuring the lunula (Figure 7.4). This discoloration, which stops suddenly 1–2 mm from the distal edge of the nail, leaves a pink area corresponding to the onychodermal band. It lies parallel to the distal part of the nail bed and may be irregular. The condition involves all nails evenly.

A variation of Terry's nail is the Morey and Burke type in which the whitening of the nail extends to the central segment with a curved leading edge. Muehrcke's bands (Figure 7.5), which are parallel to the lunula, are separated from one another, and from the lunula, by strips of pink nail. They

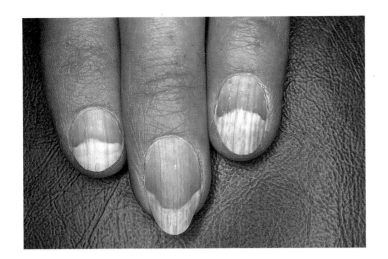

Figure 7.4

Leukonychia (apparent) due to
onycholysis.

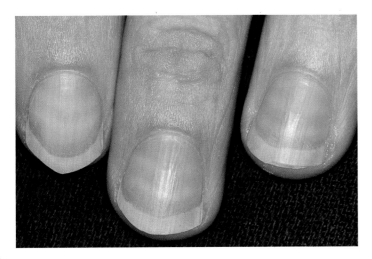

Figure 7.5

White bands due to
hypoalbuminaemia (Muehrcke's
bands).

disappear when the serum albumin level returns to normal and reappear if it falls again. It is possible that hypoalbuminaemia produces oedema of the connective tissue in front of the lunula just below the epidermis of the nail bed, changing the compact arrangement of the collagen in this area to a looser texture, resembling the structure of the lunula; hence the whitish colour. The direct correlation between the presence or disappearance of the white bands, and the serum albumin, appears to confirm this hypothesis. However, white finger nails preceded by multiple transverse white bands have been reported with normal serum albumin levels. Muehrcke's lines are common in patients undergoing systemic chemotherapy.

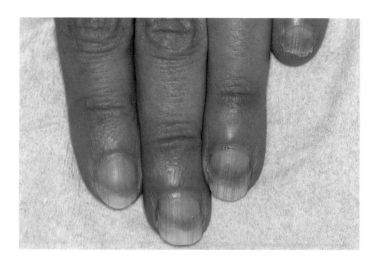

Figure 7.6

Uraemic half-and-half nail of Lindsay.

The uraemic half-and-half nail of Lindsay (Figure 7.6) consists of two parts separated more or less transversely by a well defined line; the proximal area is dull white, resembling ground glass and obscuring the lunula; the distal area is pink, reddish or brown, and occupies between 20 and 60% of the total length of the nail (average 33%). In typical cases the diagnosis presents no difficulty, but in Terry's nail the pink, distal area may occupy up to 50% of the length of the nail; under these circumstances the two types may be confused. Half-and-half nail may display a normal proximal half, the colour of the distal part being due to an increase in the number of capillaries and thickening of their walls, or melanin granules in the nail bed. Sometimes the distinctly abnormal onychodermal band extends approximately 20 to 25% from the distal portion of the finger nail as a distal crescent of pigmentation with pigment throughout the brown arc of the nail plate.

Nail changes similar to those reported by Terry, Lindsay and Muehrcke have been termed 'Neapolitan nails'; they are probably simply an old age-related phenomenon in otherwise normal individuals.

Anaemia may produce pallor of the nail (apparent leukonychia), if the haemaglobin level falls sufficiently, similar to mucous membrane and conjunctival pallor.

Dermatoses causing leukonychia

In psoriasis the nail may be affected by true leukonychia, due to involvement of the matrix, and apparent leukonychia, due to onycholysis; and by parakeratosis deposits in the nail bed. One of the earliest signs of leprosy is apparent macrolunula, which may become total in dystrophic leprosy. Leukonychia may also occur in other dermatoses, such as alopecia areata, dyshidrosis, Darier's disease and Hailey–Hailey disease (Figure 7.7). Table 7.1 is a comprehensive list of many causes and factors leading to leukonychia.

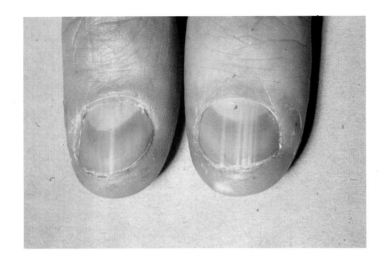

Figure 7.7

Longitudinal white lines in Hailey–Hailey disease. (Courtesy of S. Burge, UK.)

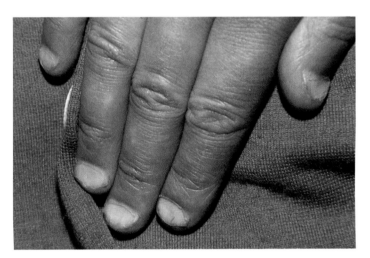

Figure 7.8

Leukokoilonychia. (Courtesy of A. Puissant, Paris)

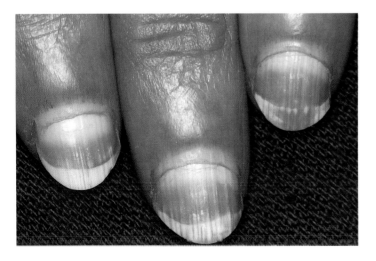

Figure 7.9

Apparent leukonychia in Raynaud's syndrome.

Table 7.1   Some causes of leukonychia

Congenital and/or hereditary
  Isolated
  Acrokeratosis verruciformis (Hopf)
  Associated with koilonychia (Figure 7.8)
  LEOPARD syndrome (lentigines,
    electrocardiographic changes, ocular
    hypertelorism, pulmonary stenosis,
    abnormalities of genitalia, retarded growth,
    deafness)
  Associated with deafness
  Leukonychia totalis, multiple sebaceous cysts,
    renal calculi
  Darier's disease – usually linear and
    longitudinal

Acquired

Pseudoleukonychia
  Diffuse form of distal and lateral subungual
    onychomycosis
  Proximal white subungual onychomycosis,
    especially in AIDS patients
  Superficial white onychomycosis
  Keratin granulation (superficial friability from
    nail varnish)
  Psoriasis

Apparent leukonychia (Figure 7.9)
  Anaemia
  Cancer chemotherapeutic agents
  Cirrhosis (Terry's sign)
  Dyshidrosis
  Half-and-half nail (renal diseases) and distal
    crescent pigmentation
  Leprosy
  Muehrcke's lines of hypoalbuminaemia

True leukonychia
  Alkaline metabolic disease
  Alopecia areata
  Carcinoid tumours of the bronchus
  Cardiac insufficiency
  Cytotoxic and other drugs (emetine,
    pilocarpine, sulphonamide, cortisone)
  Erythema multiforme
  Exfoliative dermatitis
  Fasting periods in orthodox Jews and Moslems
  Fracture
  Gout
  Hodgkin's disease
  Hypocalcaemia
  Infectious diseases and infectious fevers
  Intra-abdominal malignancies
  Kidney transplant
  Leuko-onycholysis paradentotica
  Leprosy
  Menstrual cycle
  Myocardial infarction
  Occupational
  Pellagra
  Peripheral neuropathy
  Poisoning (antimony, arsenic, fluoride, lead,
    thallium)
  Protein deficiency
  Psoriasis
  Psychotic episodes (acute)
  Renal failure (acute or chronic)
  Shock
  Sickle cell anaemia
  Surgery
  Sympathetic leukonychia
  Trauma (single or repeated)
  Tumours (benign), cysts pressing on matrix
  Ulcerative colitis
  Zinc deficiency

Table 7.2 Some causes of melanonychia

Black
    Naevi (Figure 7.10)
    Racial (Figure 7.11)
    Drugs, e.g. adriamycin, cyclophosphamide
    Haemorrhage (Figure 7.12) (*see* Chapter 9)
    Malignant melanoma (*see* Chapter 5)
    Onychomycoses (*Trichophyton rubrum
        nigricans*, dematiaceous fungi)

Brown
    Exogenous
        Drugs and dyes, e.g. dithranol, potassium
            permanganate, (Figures 7.13–7.16)
    Endogenous
        Naevi, lentigines
        Laugier–Hunziker–Baran syndrome (*see*
            Chapter 5)
        Peutz–Jeghers–Touraine syndrome
        Racial (negroid and mongoloid)
        Addison's disease
        Drugs, e.g. chlorpromazine, tetracyclines,
            ketoconazole, sulphonamides, cytotoxics,
            acyclovir
        Fetal hydantoin syndrome
        Haemochromatosis
        Malnutrition
        Nail enamels and hardeners
        Pregnancy
        Thyroid disease

Table 7.3 Some causes of LM

Idiopathic

Racial
    Dark-skinned races (negroid and mongoloid)

Systemic
    Addison's disease of the adrenal gland
    Adrenalectomy for Cushing's disease
    Carcinoma of the breast
    Drugs
    Irradiation
    Malnutrition
    Photochemotherapy
    Pregnancy
    Secondary syphilis
    Vitamin B12 deficiency

Dermatological
    Amyloid (primary)
    Basal cell carcinoma
    Bacterial infection
    Bowen's disease
    Fungal infection
    Laugier–Hunziker–Baran syndrome
    Lichen planus
    Malignant melanoma
    Peutz–Jeghers–Touraine syndrome
    Porphyria cutanea tarda
    Radiotherapy and radiodermatitis

Regional and local
    Carpal tunnel syndrome
    Repeated minor injuries
    Trauma (acute or repeated)

Melanonychia (brown/black nail)

> **An acquired single streak of LM is a melanoma until proved otherwise!**

This colour change is potentially the most serious because malignant melanoma (*see* Chapter 5) may present in many guises;

many less significant abnormalities can produce brown or black discoloration (Table 7.2). Most of the causes will be self-evident at the time of presentation, either from the history or on careful medical examination.

Bearing in mind the potential risk of malignant melanoma, one should rule out

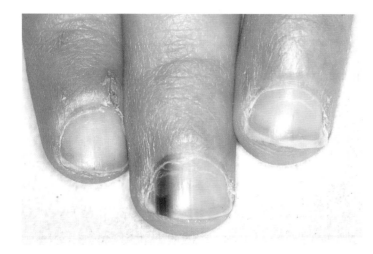

Figure 7.10

LM – congenital naevus.

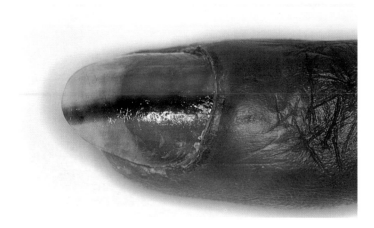

Figure 7.11

LM – acquired.

the other conditions that may present with this sign (see Table 7.3). When no specific cause is found, the following features should be considered with regard to possible malignant melanoma:

• Only one digit affected
• Linear pigmentation stopping before the free edge of the nail
• Periungual spread of the pigmentation
• Darkening of an established band

• Progressive widening of the linear streak with blurring of its border
• Aged over 50 years.

The following should also be excluded:

• Associated non-melanoma periungual pigmentation (pseudo-Hutchinson's sign)
• Single LM due to metastases of distant malignant melanoma
• Non-migratory haematoma or foreign body.

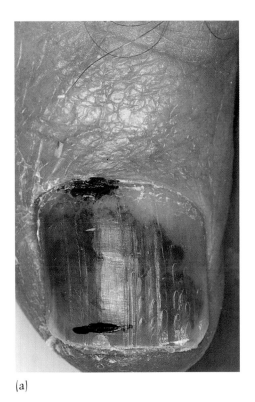

(a)

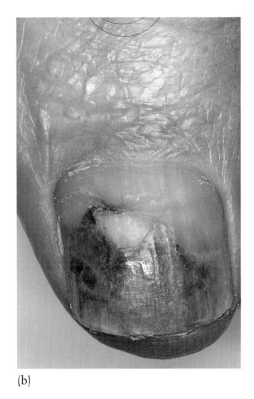

(b)

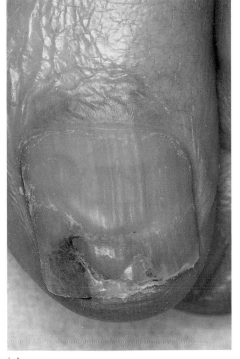

(c)

Figure 7.12

(a,b,c) Subungual haematoma showing slow resolution.

The dangers of misdiagnosis are:

- That the proper treatment of subungual melanoma will be delayed, leading to tumour spread and even death
- Treatment as for subungual melanoma will lead to over-treatment of a benign lesion and thus to unnecessary surgery. Therefore excision biopsy is crucial.

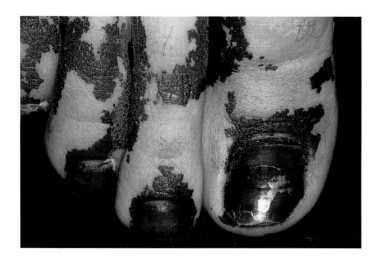

Figure 7.13

Fuchsin nail staining – Castellani's paint.

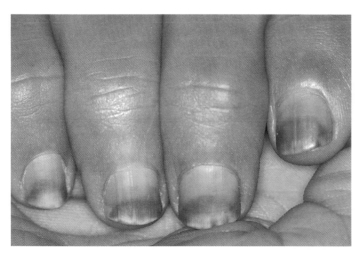

Figure 7.14

Brown staining due to henna.

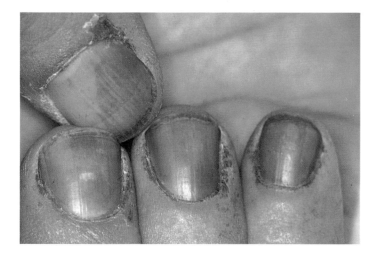

Figure 7.15

Silver nitrate staining.

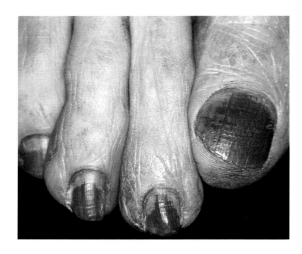

Figure 7.16

Brown staining due to potassium permanganate.

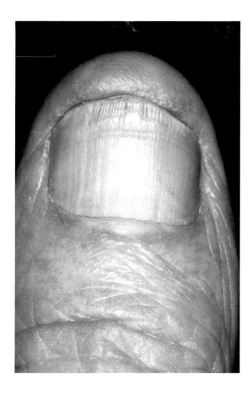

Figure 7.17

Stain due to copper in antiseptic solution.

Table 7.4   **Some causes of discoloration**

Yellow
Yellow nail syndrome (Figure 7.18)
Nail enamel and hardeners
AIDS
Carotene
Dermatophyte onychomycosis (*see* Chapter 8)
Drugs, e.g. tetracycline (fluorescent lunula),
  penicillamine, clioquinole (topical),
  mepacrine (nail bed)
Jaundice

Blue/blue-grey
Antimalarials (Figure 7.19)
Argyria
Bleomycin
Congenital pernicious anaemia
Minocycline
Phenolphthalein
Phenothiazines
Wilson's disease

Green
Aspergillus
Bullous disorders
Jaundice
'Old' haematoma (green-yellow)
Pseudomonas aeruginosa (Figure 7.20)

Red/purple
Angioma
Cirsoid aneurysm tumour
Glomus tumour (Figures 3.8, 5.25)
Congestive cardiac failure (lunula) (Figure
  7.21)
Enchodroma
Heparin (transverse)
Lichen planus
Linear red line
  Darier's disease
  Benign tumours/cysts near proximal matrix
Lupus erythematosus
Porphyria (with fluorescent light)
Rheumatoid arthritis
Warfarin

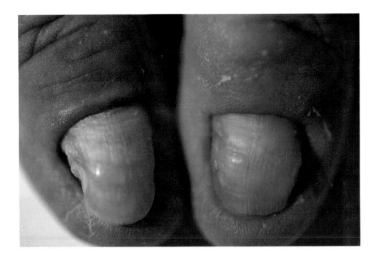

Figure 7.18
Yellow nail syndrome.

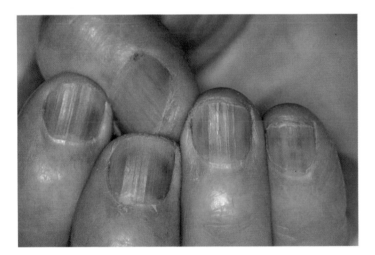

Figure 7.19
Nail discoloration due to systemic antimalarial treatment.

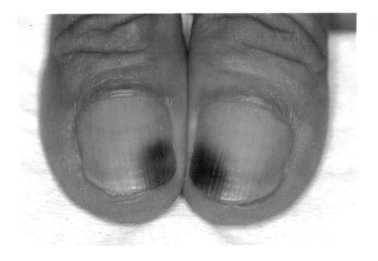

Figure 7.20
Pseudomonas colonization of onycholysis leaving nail plate pyocyanin stain.

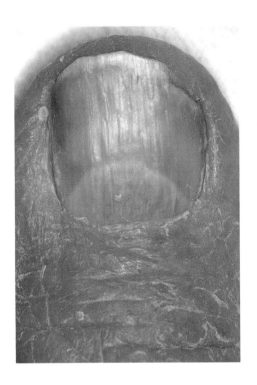

Figure 7.21

Red lunulae – occasionally seen in heart failure and alopecia areata.

Other discolorations

The variety of colour changes that may occur in the nail apparatus, other than white and brown-black, are listed in Table 7.4. Many are due to obvious cosmetic procedures, topical or oral drugs, application of antiseptics (Figure 7.17) or common diseases. None of them are of any particular significance, their presence sometimes aiding in the diagnosis of disease or pointing towards overdose of drugs.

Further reading

Melanonychia

Baran R, Haneke E (1984) Diagnostik und Therapie der streifenformigen Nagelpigmentierung, *Hautarzt* **35**: 359–365.

Baran R, Kechijian P (1989) Longitudinal melanonychia (melanonychia striata): diagnosis and management, *J Am Acad Dermatol* **21**: 1165–1175.

Other discolorations

Daniel CR III (1985) Nail pigmentation abnormalities, *Dermatol Clin* **3**: 431–443.

8 Onychomycosis and its treatment

The term onychomycosis describes the infection of the nail by fungi. Almost all cases of onychomycosis, however, result from dermatophytic invasion of the nail, onychomycosis due to non-dermatophytic moulds or yeast being relatively rare.

Onychomycosis due to dermatophytes

> **Onychomycosis is most commonly due to dermatophytes**

Three different routes of nail invasion by dermatophytic fungi were originally described by Zaias:

- Distal subungual onychomycosis
- Proximal subungual onychomycosis and
- White superficial onychomycosis

In addition, a new mode of invasion of the nail matrix by dermatophytes has recently been described: endonyx onychomycosis (EO).

In distal and lateral subungual onychomycosis (DLSO) (Figure 8.1), the most common type, dermatophytes reach the nail bed

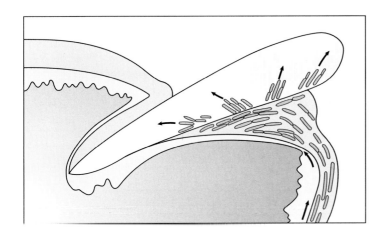

Figure 8.1

Schematic drawing of nail invasion in DLSO.

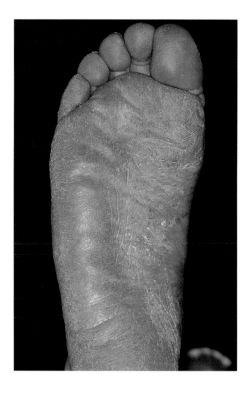

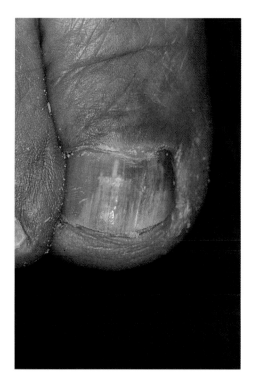

Figure 8.2

Plantar scaling due to *Trichophyton rubrum* infection in a patient with DLSO.

Figure 8.3

DLSO of the great toe: nail bed hyperkeratosis and onycholysis.

through the hyponychium. The skin of palms and soles is the primary site of infection, and plantar scaling (Figure 8.2) is usually associated with the onychomycosis. The nail bed reacts to dermatophyte invasion by becoming somewhat inflamed and hyperkeratotic. This results in subungual hyperkeratosis, the typical symptom of DLSO. Eventually, the nail plate separates from the nail bed resulting in onycholysis (Figure 8.3). In some cases the nail plate is partially absent, detached nail having been clipped by the patient (Figure 8.4). Nail destruction due

to fungal invasion of the entire thickness of the nail plate (total onychomycosis) is rare and usually takes several years to reach this stage.

Distal subungual onychomycosis is most commonly caused by *Trichophyton rubrum*. It can also be due to *T. mentagrophytes* var. interdigitale. Other dermatophytes can occasionally be responsible. It may be mostly limited to toe nails, although finger nails are less commonly affected (Figure 8.5), often presenting as the 'one hand–two foot' syndrome. When distal subungual onycho-

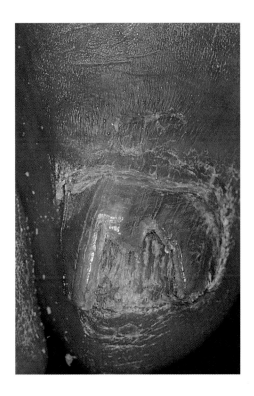

Figure 8.4

DLSO: the hyperkeratotic nail bed is evident after clipping of the detached nail plate.

mycosis involves finger nails, palmar infection with scaling is usually evident (Figure 8.6). Infection of the inguinal folds can also be observed (Figure 8.7). *Trichophyton rubrum* var. nigricans onychomycosis occasionally produces black pigmentation of the nail due to direct production of melanin-related pigment by the fungus (Figure 8.8).

In proximal subungual onychomycosis (PSO), dermatophytes reach the nail matrix keratogenous zone through the proximal nail fold horny layer (Figure 8.9). Fungal elements are typically located in the ventral nail with minimal inflammatory reaction. Proximal subungual onychomycosis presents as an area of leukonychia in the proximal portion of the nail plate (Figures 8.10a,b). The nail plate surface is normal because fungi do not penetrate the dorsal nail. This type of onychomycosis is due to *T. rubrum* and was very rare before the HIV epidemic. In the last few years it has become quite common in AIDS patients, in whom it often affects several digits concurrently.

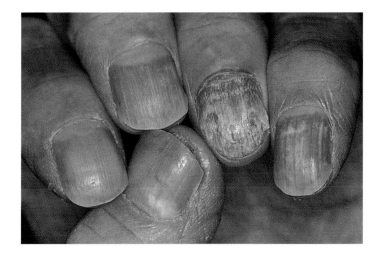

Figure 8.5

DLSO of several fingers.

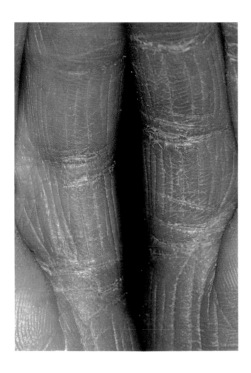

Figure 8.6

Palmar involvement in the patient of Figure 8.5.

In white superficial onychomycosis (WSO) dermatophytes colonize the most superficial layers of the nail plate without penetrating it (Figure 8.11). The nail plate surface presents small white, opaque, friable spots that represent fungal colonies in the most superficial layers of the nail plate (Figure 8.12). White superficial onychomycosis is most exclusively caused by *T. mentagrophytes* var. interdigitale and is frequently associated with Tinea pedis interdigitalis (Figure 8.13). Invasion of the superficial nail plate from *T. rubrum* var. nigricans (as well as the non-dermatophytic mould *Scytalydium dimidiatum*) is responsible for the so-called 'black superficial onychomycosis', in which the nail plate surface shows pigmented spots.

In Endonyx onychomycosis (EO) dermatophytes reach the nail plate through the plantar skin, as in DLSO (Figure 8.14). However, instead of colonizing the nail bed, fungal elements promptly invade and penetrate the nail plate. This variety of onychomycosis is associated with *T. soudanense* infection. EO produces milky-white discoloration of the nail plate without subungual hyperkeratosis and onycholysis (Figure 8.15). Plantar infection is usually evident (Figure 8.16).

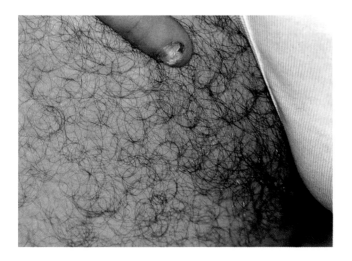

Figure 8.7

Tinea cruris in a patient affected by DLSO of several finger nails due to *Trichophyton rubrum*.

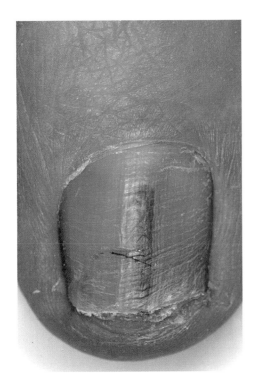

Figure 8.8

Fungal melanonychia due to *Trichophyton rubrum*.

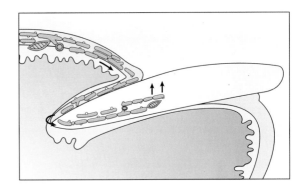

Figure 8.9

Schematic drawing of nail invasion in PSO.

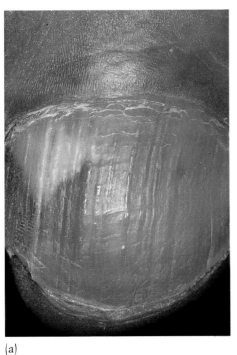

(a)

(b)

Figure 8.10

(a,b) PSO: the proximal nail shows an area of leukonychia. The nail surface is normal.

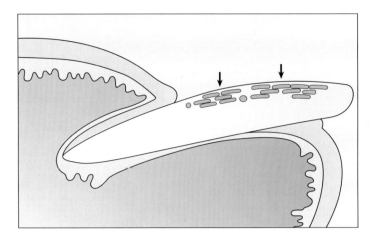

Figure 8.11

Schematic drawing of nail invasion in WSO.

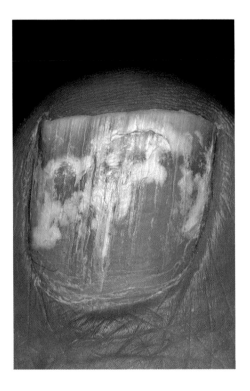

Figure 8.12

WSO: the nail plate surface presents numerous white, opaque and friable spots.

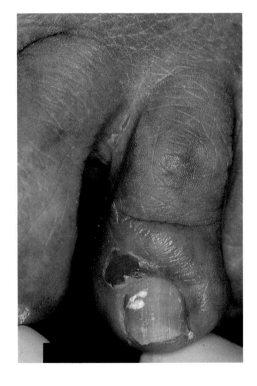

Figure 8.13

Tinea pedis interdigitalis in a patient with WSO

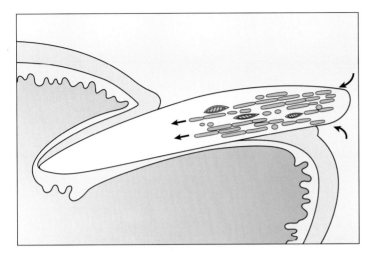

Figure 8.14

Schematic drawing of nail invasion in EO.

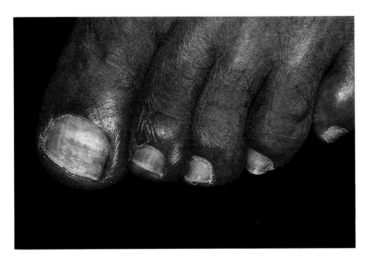

Figure 8.15

EO: milky-white discoloration of the nail plate in the absence of subungual hyperkeratosis and onycholysis.

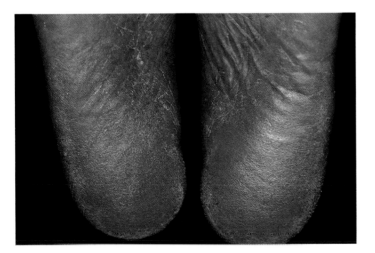

Figure 8.16

Plantar infection due to *Trichophyton soudanense* in the patient seen in Figure 8.15.

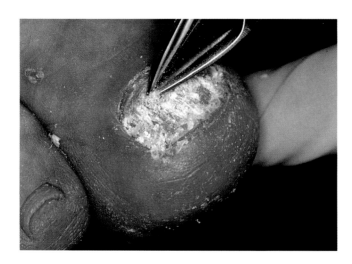

Figure 8.17

Collection of specimens in DSO. Subungual debris should be collected in the most proximal portion of the affected nail bed after clipping of the onycholytic nail plate.

Total dystrophic onychomycosis represents the most advanced form of all the types.

Diagnosis

> **Finger nail fungal infection is rare in the absence of toe nail involvement or tinea pedis**

Diagnosis of dermatophyte nail invasion can be established by the isolation and identification of the fungi from the affected nail, provided that no local or systemic antifungal has been taken recently by the patient. The site from which diagnostic specimens should be taken depends on the type of onychomycosis:

- In DLSO subungual debris should be collected from the nail bed after clipping off the overlying onycholytic nail plate

(Figure 8.17). It is very important to obtain material from the most proximal portion of the affected nail bed.
- In PSO fungi are restricted to the ventral nail plate. When the affected area is far from the distal edge of the nail, collection of the specimens requires punch biopsy of nail plate.
- In WSO the material can easily be obtained by scraping the areas of leukonychia or melanonychia from the superficial nail plate (Figure 8.18).
- In EO nail clippings contain many fungal elements and can be used directly for culture.

Direct microscopic examination of the specimens can be performed using KOH preparations. Nail debris is placed on a glass slide and a drop of a 40% KOH solution with ink (3 ml of KOH solution mixed with 1 cartridge of ink) added. After applying a cover-slip, the slide is place in a moist chamber for 2 hours to permit clearing of the keratin; it is then viewed under a microscope

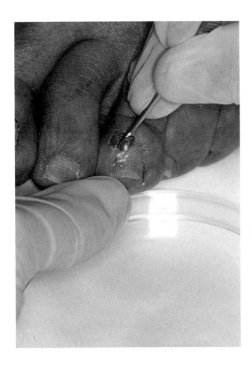

Figure 8.18

Collection of specimens in WSO. Nail debris can be obtained by scraping the areas of leukonychia on the superficial nail plate.

(Figure 8.19). A formulation of KOH and dimethylsulphoxide (DMSO) provides faster clearing of the specimen.

Cultures are performed using Sabouraud's medium with 0.05% chloramphenicol and 0.4% cycloheximide (actidione). These are incubated at 26° to 28°C for 2 to 3 weeks. Gross colony morphology (Figure 8.20) and microscropic examination of the mycelia stained with lactophenol cotton blue permit the identification of the causative dermatophyte (Figure 8.21).

Media containing a phenol red pH indicator that changes from yellow to red in the presence of dermatophytes are also available (DTM). These media contain antibiotics and cycloheximide to inhibit contaminant bacteria and fungi. However, some contaminants can still grow in the medium and produce a red discoloration that may be erroneously interpreted as a sign of dermatophyte growth. Although routine use of these media is not recommended, they can be helpful when laboratory facilities are not available.

Isolation of dermatophytes from the nails may be difficult as fungi may be scarcely viable and will not grow in cultures. Failure

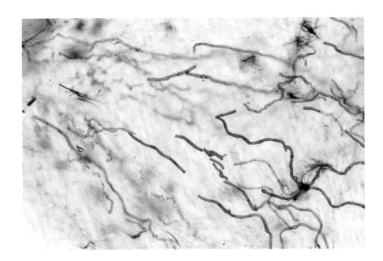

Figure 8.19

Nail preparation in 40% KOH and ink showing dermatophyte filaments.

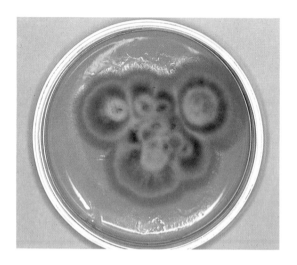

Figure 8.20

Culture of *Trichophyton rubrum* on Sabouraud's medium after 20 days' incubation at 26°C.

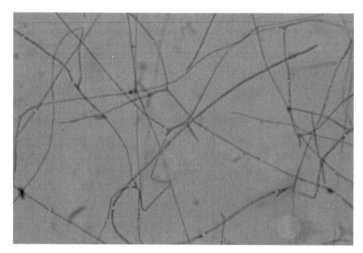

Figure 8.21

Microscopic examination of a culture of *Trichophyton soudanense* showing septate hyphae with reflexive branching and chains of arthrospores.

rate for nail culture is high (20–30%) and cultures should always be repeated when the clinical picture strongly suggests onychomycosis. Examination of material taken from associated skin lesions is advisable since these usually give profuse dermatophyte growth. In the presence of a positive skin culture, nail cultures should be repeated and a nail biopsy eventually considered if necessary.

> **Onychomycosis may be secondary to other factors – important if treatment fails!**

Differential diagnosis

Differential diagnosis between onychomycosis and psoriasis can be very difficult since subungual hyperkeratosis, onycholysis, splinter haemorrhages and diffuse nail 'crumbling' are clinical signs of both conditions. Moreover, dermatophytes or other fungi can occasionally colonize psoriatic nails, especially when the nail plate is grossly deformed. Therefore, positive culture does not exclude the diagnosis of psoriasis.

Treatment

Except for superficial onychomycosis, which can be treated with any topical antifungal agent after scraping of the affected areas, treatment of dermatophyte onychomycosis usually requires systemic antifungal therapy. However, when only the distal nail is affected and the patient's general condition makes systemic treatment questionable, since the development of the transungual drug delivery system (TUDDS) topical therapy can be tried using daily 8% ciclopirox or weekly 5% amorolfine nail lacquer. It should be continued for at least 6 months in finger nail onychomycosis and 12 months in toe nail infection – 8% ciclopirox once daily, 5% amorolfine nail lacquer once or twice weekly. A combination of bifonazole 1% in a 40% urea ointment is a possible alternative.

Until recently oral treatment of onychomycosis had consisted of two antifungal drugs: griseofulvin and ketoconazole, the latter being rarely used in recent years due to its hepatotoxicity. Treatment of onychomycosis with griseofulvin, however, requires long-term administration of the drug (6 months for finger nails, up to 18 months for toe nails), and high drug dosages (up to 2 g per day). Toe nail infection often fails to respond and recurrence is common. In the last few years three new systemic antimycotic agents have been introduced: fluconazole, itraconazole and terbinafine.

All these drugs have been shown to reach the distal nail soon after therapy is started and to persist in the nail plate for long periods (2 to 6 months) after the end of treatment. The persistence of high post-treatment drug levels in the nail allows for shorter treatment periods with fewer relapses and side-effects. Partial nail avulsion and concomitant treatment with a topical antifungal agent further reduce relapses and shortens the duration of treatment. Onychomycosis of the toe nails is more difficult to cure and recurs more frequently than onychomycosis of the finger nails.

Fluconazole and itraconazole are triazole derivatives with a broad spectrum of fungistatic activity. Itraconazole is effective at dosages of 200 mg per day for 2 to 4 months. This agent has been shown to be effective even when given as intermittent therapy (400 mg daily for 1 week every month for 3 to 6 months).

Terbinafine is an allylamine derivative with primary fungicidal properties against dermatophytes. This drug is probably more effective and safer than other antimycotics for long-term treatment of onychomycosis due to dermatophytes. Recommended dosage is 250 mg per day for 2 months (finger nails) to 4 months (toe nails). Preliminary studies show that terbinafine may also be effective at the dosage of 500 mg daily for 1 week a month (intermittent therapy).

When onychomycosis is cured it is advisable to continue application of a topical conventional antifungal on the previously affected nails, soles and toe webs to reduce the chance of relapse, unless the new transungual antifungal delivery systems (5% amorolfine and 8% ciclopirox) are used in a preventive manner.

Onychomycosis due to non-dermatophytic moulds

Onychomycosis due to non-dermatophytic moulds is rare, accounting for less than 3%

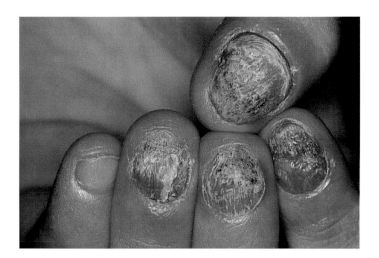

Figure 8.22

Candida onychomycosis in a child with chronic mucocutaneous candidiasis.

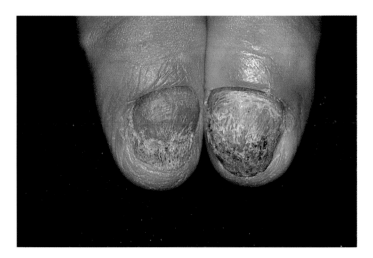

Figure 8.23

Chronic mucocutaneous candidiasis: the affected digits have a bulbous appearance with erythema and swelling of the proximal and lateral nail folds. The nail bed is hyperkeratotic and the nail plate is thickened and highly dystrophic due to diffuse crumbling. Complete destruction of the nail plate is commonly observed.

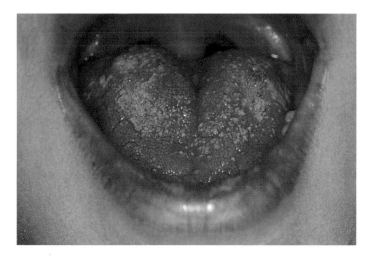

Figure 8.24

Oral candidiasis in the patient seen in Figure 8.23.

of nail infections. Moulds that have been proven to cause onychomycosis include *Scytalidium* species (*Hendersonula toruloidea*), *Scopulariopsis brevicaulis* and *Fusarium* species. The latter may produce distal subungual onychomycosis, white superficial onychomycosis and proximal subungual onychomycosis with paronychia. *Scytalydium* species and *Scopulariopsis* produce nail lesions indistinguishable from distal subungual onychomycosis. *Scytalydium dimidiatum* may also produce black superficial onychomycosis (*see* p. 158). Even though moulds can be occasionally isolated from dystrophic toe nails, their role as primitive pathogens is still unclear, as they most commonly colonize nails with pre-existing nail disease, especially dermatophytic onychomycosis or traumatic dystrophies.

Diagnosis

Diagnosis of non-dermatophytic mould nail infection requires the isolation of the fungus on direct examination of the material obtained from the suspected lesion and repeated isolation by culture of a species of fungus compatible with the finding on direct microscopic examination. In addition, cultures for dermatophytes should be regularly negative.

Since non-dermatophytic moulds are sensitive to cycloheximide and do not grow on any medium containing this antibiotic, Sabouraud's dextrose agar without cycloheximide should be used for any specimen suspected of containing these pathogens. *Scytalydium* species grow in 2 to 3 days at 26°C.

Treatment

Onychomycosis due to *Scytalidium* species is usually poorly responsive to topical and systemic treatment. Onychomycosis due to other non-dermatophytic moulds can be successfully cured by the avulsion of the affected nails.

Candida onychomycosis

> *Candida* growth from the nail is always a secondary phenomenon – due to local or systemic factors

Candida albicans can frequently be isolated from the subungual area of onycholytic nails as well as from the proximal nail fold of chronic paronychia. In both these conditions, however, *Candida* colonization is only a secondary phenomenon since topical or systemic antimycotics do not cure the nail abnormalities. Nail invasion by *Candida albicans* usually indicates an underlying immunological defect and is almost exclusively seen in chronic mucocutaneous candidiasis; in the latter, *Candida albicans* invasion of the nail plate is associated with an inflammatory reaction of the proximal nail fold, nail matrix, nail bed and hyponychium (Figure 8.22). The affected digits have a bulbous appearence with erythema and swelling of the proximal and lateral nail folds. The nail bed is hyperkeratotic and the nail plate is thickened and highly dystrophic due to diffuse 'crumbling'. Complete destruction of the nail plate is commonly observed (Figure 8.23). Oral candidiasis is present in almost all patients (Figure 8.24).

Diagnosis

The diagnosis of *Candida* nail invasion is made by culturing nail scrapings in Sabouraud's medium at 37°C. Isolated *Candida* strains should be tested for sensitivity to imidazoles.

Treatment

Nail lesions of chronic mucocutaneous candidiasis require systemic treatment. Ketoconazole (400 mg daily) and itraconazole (200 mg daily) are both effective, the latter having a safer side-effect profile.

Further reading

Baran R, Dawber RPR (1994) *Diseases of the nails and their management*, 2nd edn, (Oxford, Blackwell Scientific Publications).

Haneke E (1991) Fungal infection of the nail, *Semin Dermatol* **10**: 41–53.

Zaias N (1985) Onychomycosis, *Dermatol Clin* **3**: 445–460.

9 Traumatic disorders of the nail with special reference to the toes and painful nail

Three distinct sections will be dealt with under this heading:

1 Major trauma, involving any digit
2 Repeated microtrauma
3 The painful nail – with some deliberate overlap with sections 1 and 2.

Major trauma

This section will only consider major trauma, single overwhelming injury, necessitating only minor 'office' surgery. Complex laceration and most of the traumatic abnormalities are beyond the intended scope of this book. Damage from acute trauma may have immediate and/or delayed effects.

Haematoma

Acute subungual haematoma is usually obvious (Figures 9.1–9.3), occurring shortly after painful trauma, for example a car door slammed on fingers or a heavy object dropped on a toe nail. The blood which

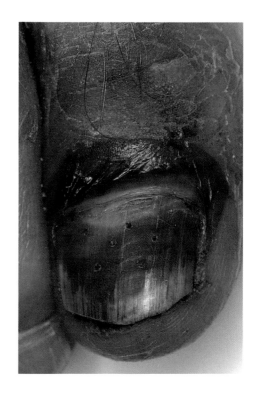

Figure 9.1

Severe traumatic haematoma.

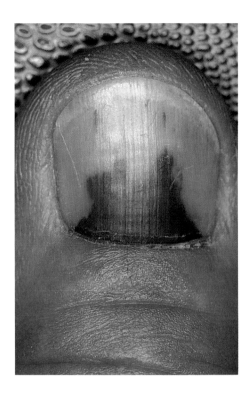

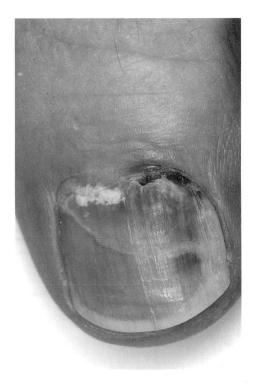

Figure 9.2

Matrix haematoma migrating distally into the nail bed.

Figure 9.3

Haematoma causing partial onychomadesis.

accumulates under the nail plate intensifies the pain which is severe. The technique used to drain the blood depends on the size of the haematoma. This prevents delay in the regrowth of the nail and secondary onychodystrophy resulting from pressure on the matrix by the accumulated blood.

Partial haematoma

Splinter haemorrhages are produced by the disruption of small vessels of the dermal ridges of the nail bed. They are more common in males than in females and in the first three fingers of each hand. With increased trauma, more dermal ridges are involved, resulting in ecchymoses. Subungual haematoma usually appears shortly after trauma, but if the injury occurs below the proximal nail fold, the haemorrhage may not be visible for 2 to 3 days. Haemorrhage in the matrix is incorporated into the nail plate; bleeding distal to the lunula remains subungual.

Total haematoma

Haematoma involving more than 25% of the visible nail is the warning sign of severe nail

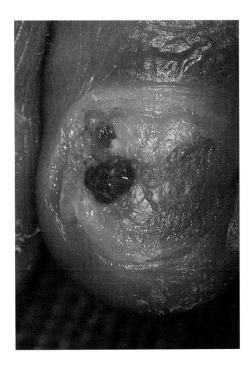

Figure 9.4

Pyogenic granuloma.

bed injury and possible underlying phalangeal fracture; an X-ray is therefore mandatory. Potential development of osteterminalisitis (infection under the nail) is a hazard, as it can spread quickly, affecting the underlying nail structures.

Nail shedding

Nail shedding may occur acutely either by direct force or following subungual haematoma; it may also appear some months after the event.

Acute paronychia

Acute paronychia may result from a penetrating thorn or splinter into the nail fold. Infection is usually painful and due to *Staphylococcus aureus*. Systemic antibiotic therapy is indicated at an early stage. If response does not occur within two days, then removal of the proximal portion of the nail plate is indicated.

Pyogenic granuloma

Pyogenic granuloma (Figure 9.4) is a benign haemangioma which typically follows skin injury. It may develop in the nail bed after a penetrating wound of the nail plate. Tenderness and a tendency to bleed easily are characteristic features. Pyogenic granuloma may be removed by excision at its base, followed by the use of aluminium chloride solution as a haemostat. Histological examination is essential to rule out amelanotic melanoma.

Delayed effects of major trauma

These are numerous (Figures 9.5–9.10). Trauma-induced Beau's line accompanied by pyogenic granuloma of the proximal nail folds of the affected fingers from trauma on the palm and the arm has been reported. Delayed effects of major trauma include permanent damage of the nail matrix, sometimes with unequal growth of different sections of the nail plate. Damage to the matrix may result in a split extending along the entire length of the nail, or a longitudinal prominent ridge, and may even result in ectopic nail due to the altered position of the matrix following the trauma. Trauma to the proximal nail fold may be responsible for pterygium formation. Longitudinal melanonychia following acute

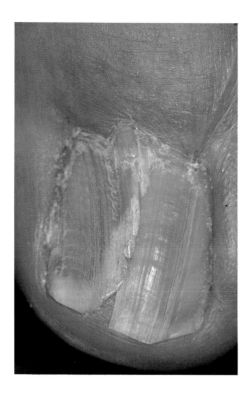

Figure 9.5

Post-traumatic fissures.

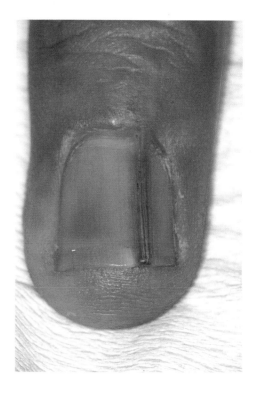

Figure 9.6

Post-traumatic nail ridge.

trauma is rare in white Caucasians. Hook nail is observed when the nail bed is shortened after distal section of the bony phalanx. Any traumatic force to the distal phalanx can result in bony changes affecting the future nail structure. An example of this is the subungual exostosis which often leads to onychocryptosis with a 'tented' hallux nail whose lateral and medial edges impinge on their corresponding nail grooves.

Significant injury was thought to be associated with the development of some cases of subungual melanoma; this is still debatable.

Repeated microtrauma of the nail apparatus

Chronic trauma implies repeated minor injury often unnoticed by the patient. A history of nail trauma as a cause of onychodystrophy can therefore be more difficult to elicit. Repeated microtrauma to the toe nail would be of little importance were it not for the shoes of the fashion conscious women and for their significance to the athlete and to the elderly where faulty

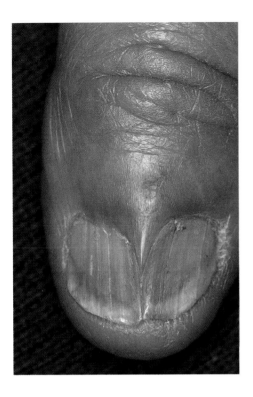

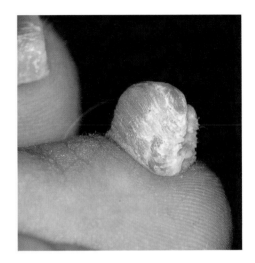

Figure 9.7

Post-traumatic nail dystrophy – pterygium scar.

Figure 9.8

Post-traumatic hyperkeratosis.

ambulatory biomechanics play a prominent role. Finally, congenital or acquired abnormalities of the foot may lead to a variety of foot and nail hyperkeratotic problems.

In the older age groups, women outnumber men in developing chronic foot disorders, for example with double the number of ingrowing toe nails. Women's fashion shoes cause far more deformed 'lesser' toes. Inappropriate footwear often starts in childhood. A UK study of 9-year-old children's feet found that 25% of girls compared with 1% of boys wear unsuitable shoes, notably a too narrow toebox. Improper fitting often continues into adult life, with women consistently wearing shoes that are 'smaller than their feet'.

Toe nail problems in the aged can be particularly distressing. Not only are they complicated by reduced circulation, with all the dangers to the foot that this can entail, but poor eyesight and decreased manual dexterity in the elderly patient contribute to nail management difficulties. In addition, sensation in the feet may be diminished and the reduced mobility in the joints of the lower extremity makes it difficult to place

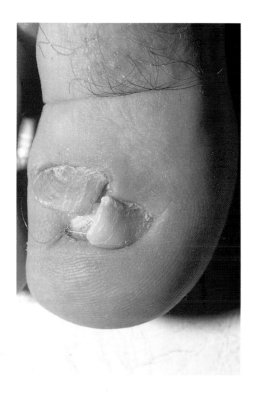

Figure 9.9

Traumatic matrix distortion and nail plate dystrophy – ectopic nail.

the foot in a convenient position for nail care.

Poorly fitting shoes and/or abnormal biomechanics have in common abnormalities of the gait cycle (heel strike, stance phase, and push-off) (*see* Chapter 1). Hallux nail pathology appears to be the most common functional and traumatic disorder. This is due to forces that can be divided into three body planes:

- Transverse plane changes (hallux valgus) (Figure 9.11). This deformity may cause pronounced changes in the nail apparatus including hyperkeratosis of the tibial nail fold and the distal medial subungual area; recalcitrant ingrowing toe nail with granulation tissue in the lateral nail groove and adjacent bed of the great toe; lateral deviation of the big toe nail resulting in lateral pincer nail and laterally 'wound' screw-shaped onychogryphosis.
- Frontal plane changes (adding proximal bony instabilities).
- Sagittal plane changes that clinically raise or dorsiflex the digit.

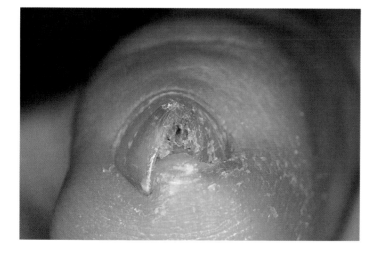

Figure 9.10

'Tented' nail over a bony exostosis.

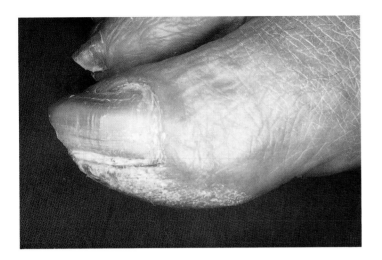

Figure 9.11

Nail dystrophy due to hallux valgus. (Courtesy of B. Schubert.)

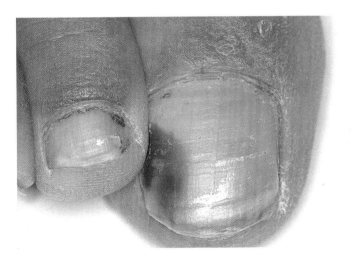

Figure 9.12

'Primary' onycholysis due to pressure from the second toe.

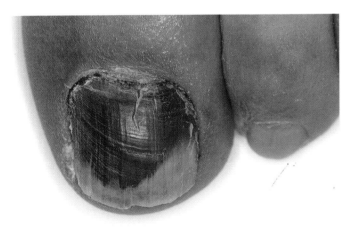

Figure 9.13

Subungual haematoma due to pressure and rubbing from the shoe toe box.

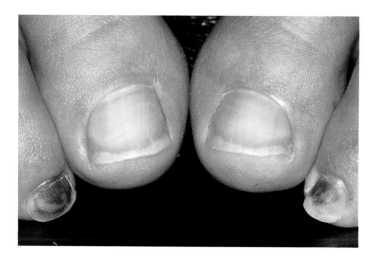

Figure 9.14

Sportsman's toe – subungual haemorrhage of second toes.

The lesser digits are most commonly affected by muscular imbalances between the extensor and flexor muscle group, producing hammer, claw or mallet toe deformities.

Alteration of the surrounding tissue

Subungual haemorrhage

Tennis (or sportman's) toe is a brown-black discoloration due to subungual haemorrhage caused by special stresses on the longest toe (great toe and/or the second toe) (Figures 9.12–9.14). Pain is associated with the appearance of the damage. In tennis, this occurs because the player frequently stops abruptly; the forward motion of the body propels the toes into the toe box and tip of the footwear. Hard playing surfaces contribute to the injury.

In distinction to tennis toe, jogger's toe tends to involve the third, fourth and fifth toes, apparently due to the constant pounding of the foot on the running surface. The process begins with erythema, oedema and onycholysis or subungual haemorrhage. Throbbing pain often accompanies this condition. Secondary infection resulting in cellulitis and abscess formation may be a rare complication.

Subungual purpura or subungual haemorrhage is often precipitated in patients with other contributory factors, for example in those taking drugs such as aspirin.

Hyperkeratotic changes

Hyperkeratoses are likely to develop when one or more of the following occur:

- Abnormal gait
- Wearing of tight shoes
- Osteoarthritis.

The frictional forces that occur between a tight shoe and a large arthritic 'condyl' in a patient with abnormal gait cause hyperkera-

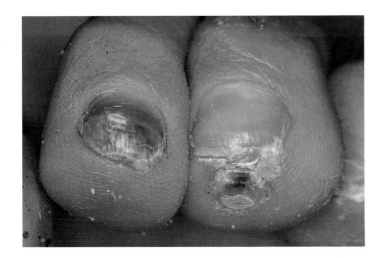

Figure 9.15

Subungual corn (heloma).

totic lesions to form first and then a corn to supervene. The corn is a modified callus with a central hard whitish parakeratotic core, often visible only after paring (Figure 9.15). When a corn of the fifth toe is seen (Figure 9.16) it may also be noted at the junction of the lateral and posterior nail fold of this toe nail. As the toe becomes hammer-shaped a painful callus occasionally develops under the pulp of the toe just below the end of the nail (end corn).

Subungual clavus or heloma, when present (Figure 9.17), usually involves the hallux toe nail and is associated with subungual exostosis or is due to some related shoe pressure from the toe box with an extended hallux. An X-ray should be taken to confirm any bony abnormality, including changes in the tufted end of the phalanx (Figure 9.18). Pressure should be eliminated with tube foam lamb's wool and by the use of a higher toe box. An emollient such as urea 20% can be useful.

The appearance of hyperkeratotic tissue in varying degrees on the lateral nail folds or in the lateral nail grooves, in response to repeated trauma, is common. It produces

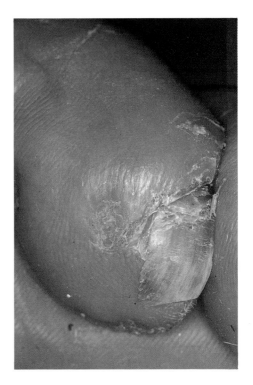

Figure 9.16

Large heloma.

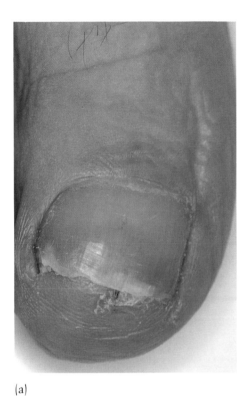

(a)

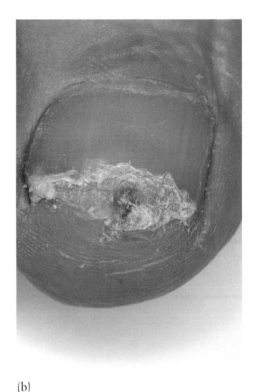

(b)

Figure 9.17

Subungual corn: (**a**) nail intact; (**b**) nail plate
clipped away to show the heloma.

pain and discomfort. This horny growth,
diffuse or localized, called onychophosis,
involves mainly the great (Figure 9.19) and
fifth toes. Management includes debridement of the hyperkeratotic tissue, thinning
of the nail plate, use of emollients to both
hydrate and lubricate the nail grooves, nail
packing to help reduce trauma and removal
of external pressure.

Various orthopaedic devices may be used
to reduce pressure and repeated microtrauma. They provide both weight diffusion
and weight dispersion. These include devices
made of felt, foam rubber, sponge rubber,
plastic as well as newer products such as
plastazote, PPT, Spenco and Sorbothane.

Onycholysis and onychomadesis

Excess friction between the nail and the shoe
may result in onycholysis and even in fluid
filled blisters (Figure 9.20). These subungual
bullae can sometimes be haemorrhagic.
Similar friction at the base of the nail may
produce onychomadesis (Figure 9.21).

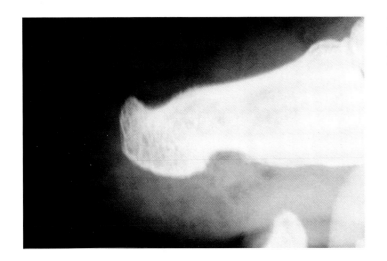

Figure 9.18

Toe X-ray showing a dorsal hyperostosis.

Separation of the nail from the subungual tissue is often seen in ballet dancers who dance on 'points' and in footballers.

Subungual hyperkeratosis is usually associated with excessive pressure and related onycholysis, and occasionally onychomycosis, especially in the elderly. Overlapping of the second toe on the lateral aspect of the hallux may also produce onycholysis in this area with or without haemorrhage.

Onychocryptosis

Four major types can be described in adults:

- Distal nail embedding
- Pincer nail
- Juvenile ingrowing toe nail
- Hypertrophy of the lateral lip

Distal nail embedding (Figure 9.22–9.24). In the great toe, a distal wall may develop after nail shedding following subungual haemorrhage, for example in tennis toe or after nail avulsion (Figure 9.22). Normally, the nail

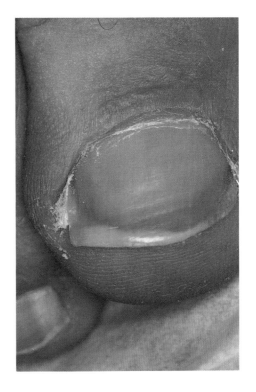

Figure 9.19

Painful lateral hyperkeratosis (from repeated microtrauma) – onychophosis.

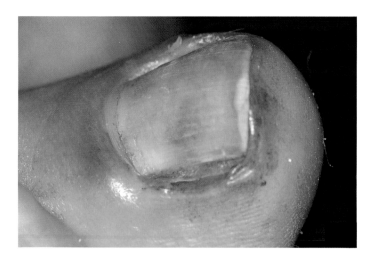

Figure 9.20

Traumatic onycholysis following bulla formation.

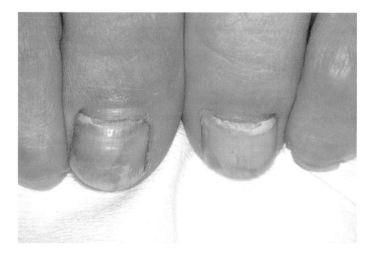

Figure 9.21

Traumatic onychomadesis.

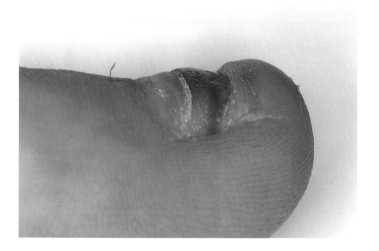

Figure 9.22

Distal nail embedding – overgrowth of distal soft tissue after nail loss. New nail may penetrate into this.

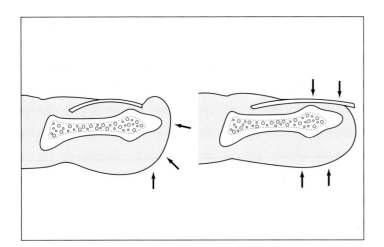

Figure 9.23

Diagram demonstrating anchoring of acrylic sculptured nail to inhibit embedding.

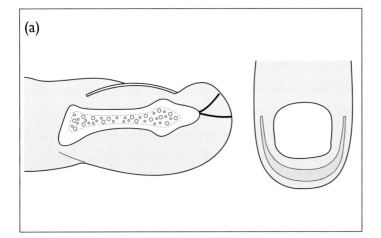

(a)

Figure 9.24

(a,b) Diagrams to show operation to remove overgrown distal soft tissue. See text for details.

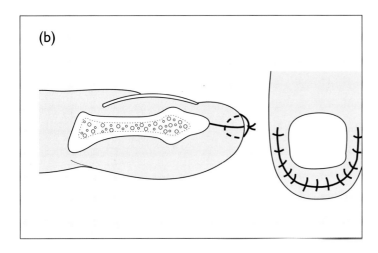

(b)

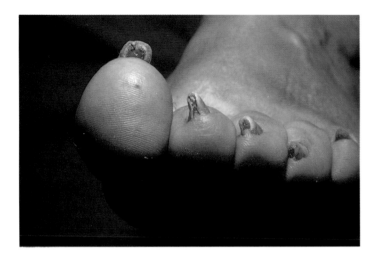

Figure 9.25

Pincer nail deformity with symmetrical involvement of several toes.

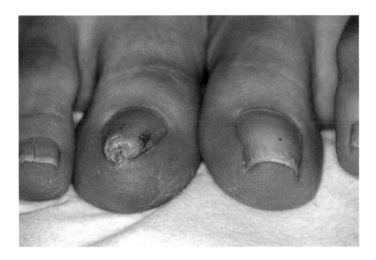

Figure 9.26

Trumpet nail – often painful.

plate position counteracts the forces that are exerted during walking. Due to lack of counterpressure, the plantar portion of the hallux pulp becomes distorted dorsally when the foot rolls up and the body weight presses on the tip of the big toe during walking. The distal wall interferes with the growth of the newly formed nail. The anchoring of an acrylic sculptured nail on the stump nail may enable it to overgrow the heaped-up distal tissue (Figure 9.23). Should this procedure not be effective a crescent-shaped wedge excision becomes necessary (Figure 9.24). A fish mouth incision is carried out parallel to the distal groove around the tip of the toe, starting and ending 3 to 5 mm proximal to the end of the lateral nail fold. A second incision is then made to yield a wedge of 4 to 8 mm at its greatest width; it has to be dissected from the bone.

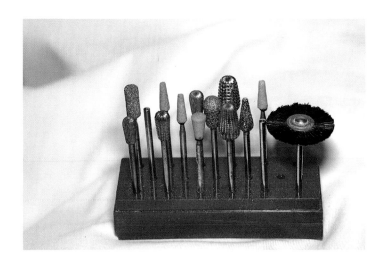

Figure 9.27

Burr equipment to remove excessive nail plate tissue. (Courtesy of S. Goettmann.)

Pincer nail (trumpet nail, omega nail, convoluted nail) (Figures 9.25, 9.26). Pincer nail is a dystrophy characterized by transverse overcurvature increasing along the longitudinal axis of the nail and reaching its greatest extent at the distal part (*see also* page 53). The edges constrict the nail bed tissue and dig into the lateral nail grooves. Pain, which is usually not too severe, may sometimes be excruciating. On occasion, pain may develop specifically under the mid-point of the distal nail edge, dorsal to the distal phalangeal tuft. Two varieties of overcurvature can be described:

1   Symmetrical involvement of several toes, usually with lateral deviation of the long axis of the hallux nail and medial deviation of the lesser toe nails. This variety is probably genetically determined. The pincer nail syndrome includes gryphosis of finger and toe nails in combination with acro-osteolytic shortening of the terminal phalanx and destructive arthrosis of the distal joints of the digits. X-ray examination reveals a wider base of the terminal phalanx, often with lateral osteophytes. Hyperostosis is frequently observed on the dorsal tuft of the distal phalanx, due to traction of the heaped-up nail bed which is firmly attached to the bone by collagen fibres.

2   Asymmetrical involvement of the halluces, the major cause being foot deformities and osteoarthritis.

Conservative management: mild cases may be improved by clipping down the lateral edge of the inward distorted nail plate, grooving the nail with a burr (Figure 9.27) extending forwards from the lunula and terminating at the free edge, and orthonyx, a nail brace technique (Figure 9.28), which is based on maintaining tension on the nail plate with the wire. Fraser's method consists of a brace constructed to fit the curved plate exactly; at one selected point a minute 'adjustment' (a slight bend) is then made to the brace and it is fitted to the plate. As the nail plate is weaker than the stainless wire, the nail plate conforms to the brace. In the months that follow, a series of 'adjustments' are made and

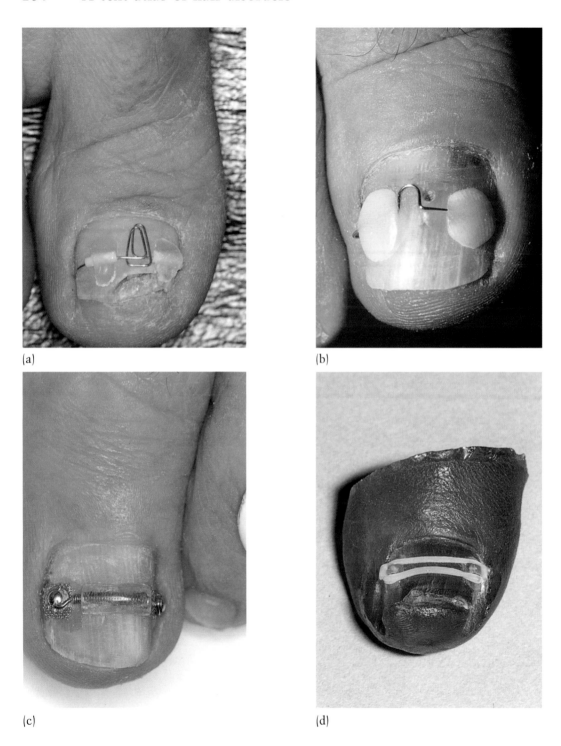

(a)

(b)

(c)

(d)

Figure 9.28

(a–d) Nail brace technique for pincer nail deformity.

almost imperceptibly the curvature decreases. Some improvements to this technique have been suggested, such as the use of brackets adapted on the dorsum of the nail and linked by a rubber band or attachment of a plastic brace on the surface of the nail. In these cases the nail plate is first flattened with an electrically driven dermatological grinder, and pliant braces are stuck transversely on the nail to counteract the overcurvature. However, the pathogenesis of pincer nail is such that all these methods are unable to give high cure rates.

The definitive procedure is said to be Haneke's surgical treatment (Figure 9.29): using a bloodless field a lateral nail strip involving one or both sides is freed from the proximal nail fold, nail bed and matrix with a Freer septum elevator, then cut longitudinally and extracted. This permits the destruction of the lateral matrix horns by phenol. The distal two-thirds of the nail is removed, then a longitudinal median incision of the nail bed is carried down to the bone. The entire nail bed is dissected from the phalanx and the dorsal tuft removed with a bone rongeur. The nail bed is spread and sutured with 6-0 PDS atraumatic sutures and kept in this position by using reversed tie-over sutures that pull the lateral nail folds apart; these are left in for 18 to 21 days. Daily povidone iodine antisepsis prevents infection.

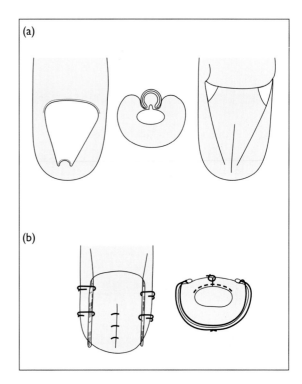

Figure 9.29

(a, b) Diagrams illustrating Haneke's technique to correct pincer nail deformity. See text for details.

Juvenile ingrowing toenail (subcutaneous ingrowing nail) (Figure 9.30). Ingrowing toe nail is created by impingement of the nail plate onto the dermal tissue of the lateral nail fold. This often results from improper trimming of the nail. Consequently, a lacerating spicule of the nail pierces the soft tissue surrounding the side of the nail, acting as a foreign body and producing inflammation with pain from perforation of the nail groove epithelium.

Conservative treatment: in mild cases, under local anaesthesia, removal of the spicule and separation of the offending nail edge from the adjacent soft tissue with a wisp of absorbent cotton coated with collodion gives immediate relief from pain. After the toe is cured, the nail must be cut square and the sharp corners smoothed away with an emery board. Unfortunately, as conservative management requires a high degree of compliance, recurrences are frequent. Sometimes, the nail groove becomes involved along its entire length by excess granulation tissue which may extend beneath the nail and overlap its dorsal

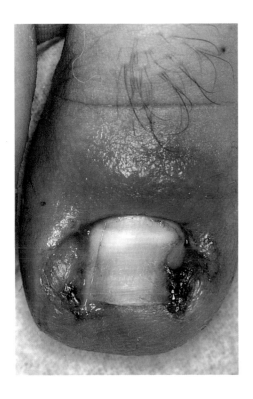

Figure 9.30

Ingrowing toe nail with chronic granulation tissue formation.

aspect. Infection is always present and pus exudes from the nail groove.

The definitive procedure calls for selective matrix horn removal which permanently narrows the nail. A lateral nail strip is freed from the proximal nail fold, nail bed and matrix with a Freer septum elevator then cut longitudinally and extracted. Using a bloodless field, this partial nail avulsion may be immediately followed by phenol cauterization. Post-operative pain is minimal since phenol has local anaesthetic action and is also antiseptic. The matrix epithelium is sloughed off and there is usually slight oozing for 2 to 4 weeks. Daily foot baths with povidone iodine soap minimize the risk of infection and accelerate healing.

Hypertrophy of the lateral lip (Figure 9.31). Hypertrophic lateral nail fold usually accompanies long-standing ingrowing nails. The nail looks normal but the soft tissue lip overgrows the nail plate. Inflammation occurs deep into the hypertrophied tissue.

Treatment consists in narrowing the nail by cauterization of the lateral horn of the nail matrix. This may be associated with an

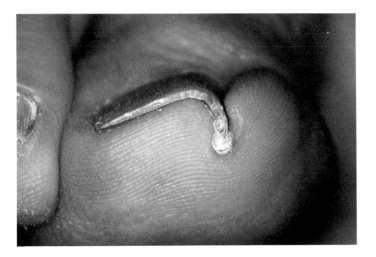

Figure 9.31

Hypertrophy of the lateral lip (nail fold).

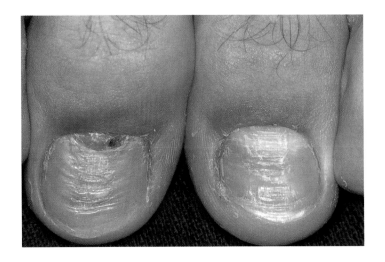

Figure 9.32

Self-induced transverse ridges/furrows.

elliptical wedge of tissue taken from the lateral wall of the toe and its distolateral portion. Complete removal of the hypertrophic lateral nail fold is a good alternative. It is followed by a transposition flap of the nail wall.

Hang nails (see *page 93*)

Hang nails often result from self-inflicted trauma. Usually limited to the hands, these consist of a small portion of horny epidermis that has split away from the lateral nail fold. They can be painful and lead to secondary bacterial infection. Although frequently found in nail biters, they can also arise from other forms of injury. Cuticle biting and picking may result in recurrent attacks of paronychia.

Paronychia of the toes

Inflammation of the nail folds is common in athletes and is characterized by swelling, erythema, pain and purulent discharge. It is

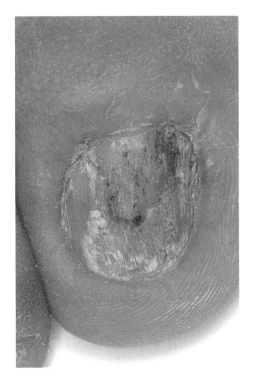

Figure 9.33

Onychotillomania of the great toe.

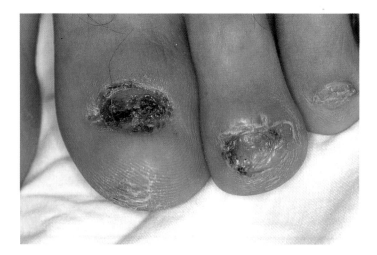

Figure 9.34

Nail dystrophy – self-damage.

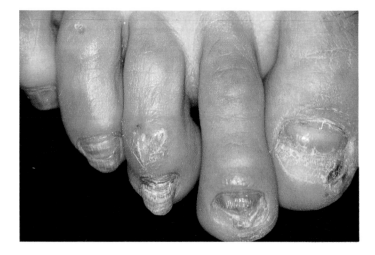

Figure 9.35

Nail shedding in a long distance runner.

often caused by pressure from the shoe or by secondary infection from ingrowing toe nail. The big toe is more often affected than the lesser toes.

Turf toe is a variant of this condition described in competitors who play on artificial turf surfaces; they rarely develop painful erythema and swelling, mainly of the great toe.

Alteration of the nail itself

This category includes:

1   Self-inflicted injury (Figures 9.32–9.34):
    • By the habit of pushing back the cuticle (*see* Chapter 2).
    • Heller's median nail dystrophy (*see* Chapter 2).

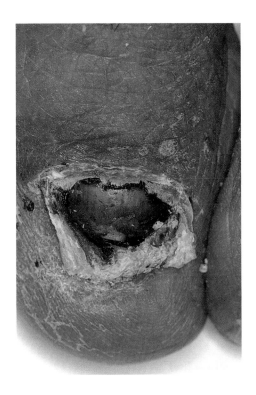

Figure 9.36

Dystrophy due to chronic shoe rubbing.

- Nail biting and picking.
- Self-inflicted nail damage may cause LM.
- Nail artifacts, caused by deliberate acts of injury to the nail apparatus with the intention of creating a 'diversion for personal gain'; they may also be caused 'subconsciously'. Nail artifacts take various forms. Such patients usually have psychological problems.

2 Nail shedding (Figure 9.35):
- Self-inflicted anonychia of the toe nails is associated with small or absent nails and crushing due to traumatic bleeding.
- Periodic shedding of the nails can result from biomechanical causes and is frequently seen in runners.

3 Worn-down nail (Figures 9.36, 9.37) (*see* Chapter 2):
- Koilonychia (toes of rickshaw boys).

4 Brittle nails (*see* Chapter 6).

5 Onychogryphosis and hypertrophic nail (*see* Chapter 4).

6 Frictional melanonychia (Figure 9.38):

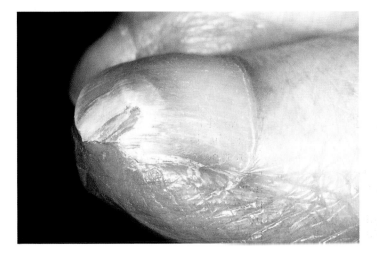

Figure 9.37

Dystrophy from shoe pressure.

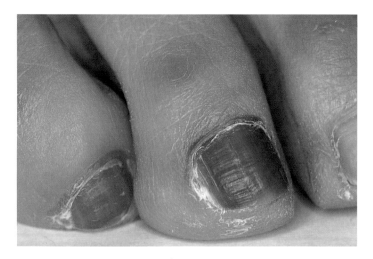

Figure 9.38

Frictional melanonychia.

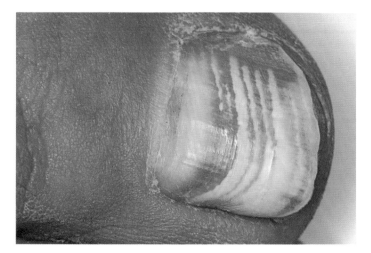

Figure 9.39

Transverse leukonychia from distal pressure on untrimmed nail.

- Frictional melanonychia of the toes can be initiated by repeated trauma from footwear.
- Friction and pressure are responsible for LM with pseudo-Hutchinson's sign in boxers.

7 Multiple transverse leukonychia (Figure 9.39). Multiple transverse white bands separated by normal pink nail and paralleling the distal shape of the lunula results from repeated microtrauma. These appear in patients with marked visible free margins of the involved toe nails (usually the big toe or the second toe when longer) indicating a lack of trimming and impinging on the distal part of the shoe.

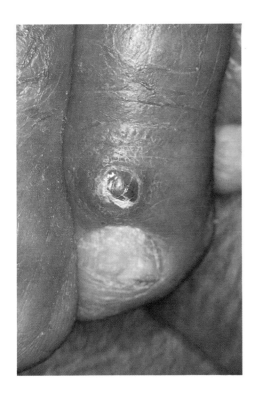

Figure 9.40

Myxoid cyst associated with distal interphalangeal joint osteoarthritis.

Alteration of the bony phalanx (see p 108)

Exostosis can be observed in ballet dancers and football players.

Alteration of the distal joint and tendon sheath (see p 108)

Mucous pseudo-cyst (Figure 9.40) can be caused by systemic conditions that affect joints and in particular the distal joint. This tumour can produce pressure on the nail matrix resulting in a longitudinal nail groove. When the second toe is longer than the other toes, it may cause increased pressure on the toe from the shoes, especially in tennis players. Treatment usually consists of removal of the cyst and overlying skin and debridement of the arthritic distal interphalangeal joint. Magnetic resonance imaging (MRI) demonstrates the relationship of the cyst to the other soft tissue structures of the toe (Figure 9.41).

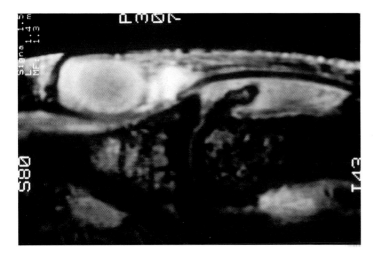

Figure 9.41

MRI scan to show myxoid pseudocyst in a second toenail in relation to other soft tissue structures. (Courtesy of A. Salon, Paris)

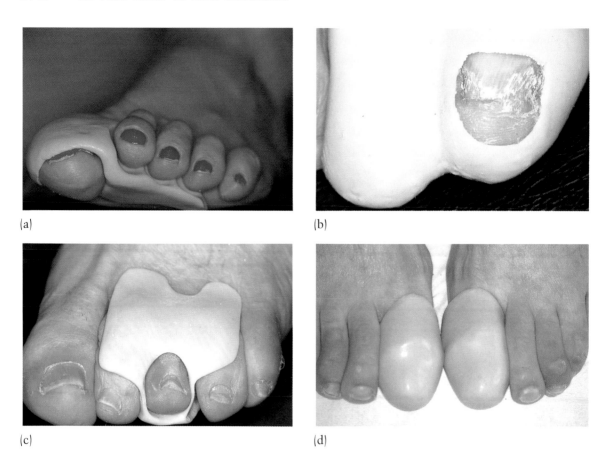

(a)

(b)

(c)

(d)

(e)

Figure 9.42

(a–h) Various shoe inserts to prevent dystropy from pressure between adjacent toes.

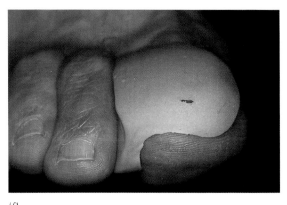

(f)

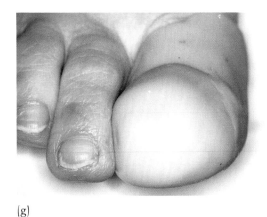

(g)

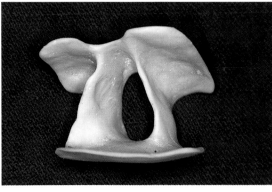

(h)

The painful nail

Pain is a non-specific and common symptom of many conditions of the nail apparatus (see Table 9.1; Figures 9.42–9.49). Apart from various forms of trauma, many inflammatory and vascular diseases may cause pain; however, pain is so subjective and inconstant a symptom that even diseases commonly known as being particularly painful may follow a rather asymptomatic course and vice versa. The entire distal phalanx, especially the finger pulp, is richly innervated. Each 'space-occupying' process, whether inflammatory or neoplastic, may produce pain because the subungual tissue consists of dense fibrous tissue closely adherent to the bone and without the 'elastic' pad of subcutaneous fat. Inflammatory conditions and tumours are squeezed in this firm subungual tissue between the hard nail plate and hard bone; slowly enlarging processes may lead to clubbing and pressure-induced bone erosion. Pain is therefore to be expected under these conditions. In addition, the tumour itself may be inherently painful, as for example with the glomus tumour. If pain subsequent to simple trauma or acute

Table 9.1   Some causes of painful nail

Trauma	Childhood malalignment
	Cold injury
	Common type
	Crush and squeeze injuries
	Ingrowing toe nail
	Splinters/foreign bodies
	Sportsman, sports shoes injuries
Inflammation	Acro-osteolysis
	Acute (and chronic) paronychia
	Dorsolateral fissures
	Gout
	Herpes simplex
	Implantation epidermoid cyst
	Osteomyelitis
	Pincer nail – severe form enclosing bone
	Post-cryosurgery – may be prolonged bone pain
	Prosector's wart (TB)
	Sarcoid dactylitis
	Subcutaneous abscess
	Subungual foreign body
	Ventral pterygium
Tumours (soft tissue and bone)	Aneurysmal bone cyst
	Bowen's disease
	Enchondromas
	Fibromas
	Glomus tumour
	Keratoacanthoma
	Leiomyoma
	Metastases
	Myxoid cyst
	Osteoid osteoma
	Osteoma, exostosis
	Secondary infection – slow-growing tumour
	Some neuromas
	Squamous cell carcinoma
	Subungual corn
	Subungual papilloma – incontinentia pigmenti
	Subungual wart
Vascular	Acute ischaemia
	Chilblains
	Raynaud's phenomenon/disease
	Rheumatoid vasculitic lesions
	Systemic sclerosis

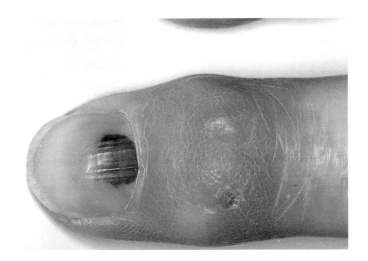

Figure 9.43

Recurrent herpes simplex with subungual haemorrhage.

inflammation does not respond to adequate therapy, either an X-ray or biopsy or both should be performed to rule out a malignant tumour. X-rays may be difficult to interpret, especially in the elderly with degenerative arthritis, and it may be necessary to repeat the X-rays or other imaging techniques if the disease does not follow the expected course, or fails to respond to treatment. Ultrasound and magnetic resonance imaging (MRI) may be useful tools but the latter is very expensive.

Further reading

Balkin SW (1993) What do women want: comfy shoes – sometimes, *JMA* **269**: 215.

Baran R (1987) Frictional longitudinal melanonychia: a new entity, *Dermatologica* **174**: 280–284.

Baran R (1990) Nail biting and picking as a possible cause of longitudinal melanonychia, *Dermatologica* **181**: 126 128.

Baran R (1995) Transverse leuconychia of toenails due to repeated microtrauma, *Br J Dermatol* **133**: 267–269.

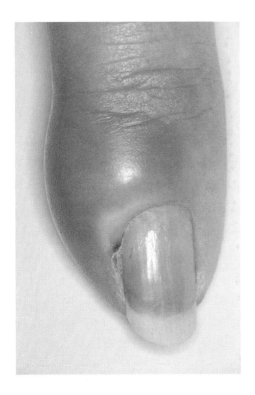

Figure 9.44

Acute paronychia.

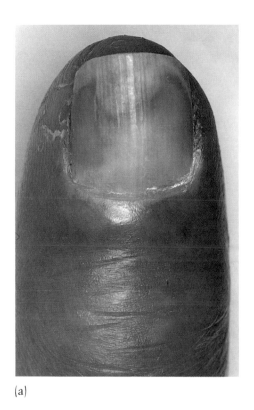

(a)

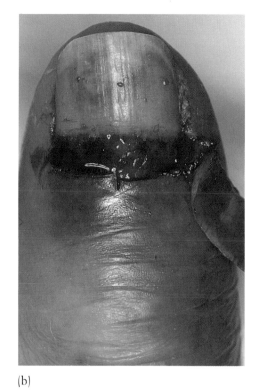

(b)

Figure 9.45

(a) Acute paronychia with pus tracking into the nail bed; (b) treatment by transverse section of the nail plate.

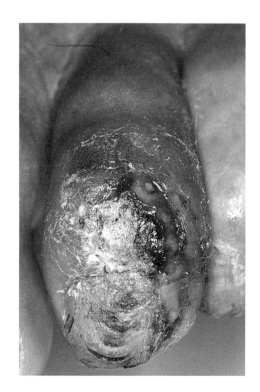

Figure 9.46

Radiodermatitis and radionecrosis of the bony phalanx following treatment of epidermal carcinoma.

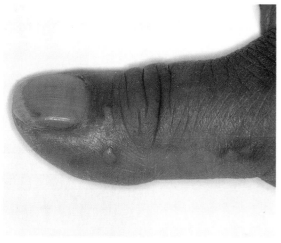

Figure 9.47

Herpes zoster.

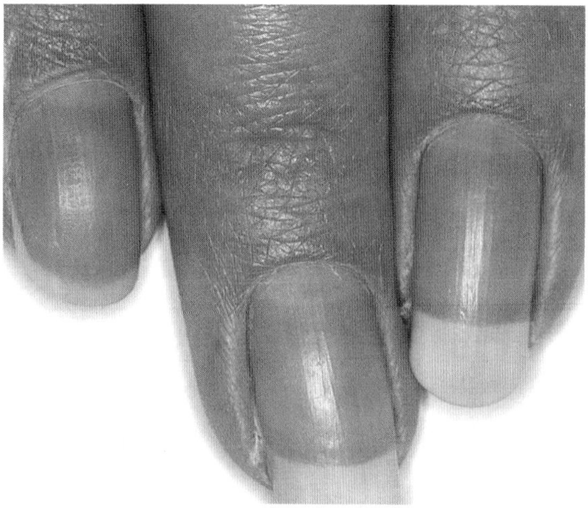

Figure 9.49

Glomus tumour.

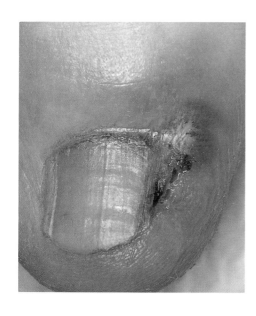

Figure 9.48

Implantation cyst following surgical treatment for ingrowing toe nail.

Baran R, Badillet G (1982) Primary onycholysis of the big toenail: review of 113 cases, *Br J Dermatol* **106**: 529–534.

Bayerl C, Moll I (1993) Longitudinal melanonychia with Hutchinson's sign in a boxer, *Hautarzt* **44**: 476–479.

Dagnall C (1976) The development of nail treatments, *Br J Chiropody* **41**: 206–207.

Doller J, Strother S (1978) Turf toe, *J Am Podiatr Assoc* **68**: 512–514.

Effendy I, Ossowski B, Happle R (1993) Zangennagel, *Hautarzt* **44**: 800–802.

Eiscle SA (1994) Conditions of the toenails, *Orthop Clin North Am* **25**: 183–187.

Fabry H (1983) Haut- und Nagelveränderungen bei Hallux valgus, *Akt Derm* **9**: 77–79.

Gibbs RC (1985) Toenail disease secondary to poorly fitting shoes or abnormal biomechanics, *Cutis* **36**: 399–400.

Gibbs RC, Boxer MC (1989) Abnormal biomechanics of feet and their cause of hyperkeratoses, *J Am Acad Dermatol* **6**: 1061–1069.

Haneke E, Baran R (1994) In: *Nail surgery and traumatic abnormalities*, eds Baran R, Dawher

RPR (Oxford, Blackwell Scientific Publications), pp. 344–415.

Helphand AE (1989) Nail and hyperkeratotic problems in the elderly foot, *AFP* **39**: 101–110.

Hurley PT, Balu V (1982) Self inflicted anonychia, *Arch Dermatol* **118**: 956–957.

Jahss MH (1979) Geriatric aspects of the foot and ankle. In: *Clinical geriatrics*, ed. Rossman I (Philadelphia, JB Lippincott) pp. 638–650.

Johnson EW, In Tarara EL (1970) Ingrown toenail: a problem among the aged, *Post Grad Med* 199–202.

O'Toole EA, Stephens R, Young MM *et al* (1995) Subungual melanoma: a relation to direct injury? *J Am Acad Dermatol* **33**: 525–528.

Price MA, Bruce S, Waidhofer W *et al* (1994) Beau's lines and pyogenic granulomas following hand trauma, *Cutis* **54**: 246–249.

Rzonca EC, Lupo PJ (1989) Pedal nail pathology: biomechanical implications, *Clin Podiatr Med Surg* **6**: 327–337.

Scher RK (1978) Jogger's toe, *Int J Dermatol* **17**: 719–720.

Stone OJ, Mullins JF (1963) The distal course of nail matrix hemorrhage, *Arch Dermatol* **88**: 186.

Zook EG (1986) Complications of the perionychium, *Hand Clin* **2**: 407–427.

10 Treatment of common nail disorders

The human nail, chemically similar to horn and hoof, is not essential for the survival of *Homo sapiens*, but it has many important functions that are crucial for the efficient use of the hands and feet. The nail is a prime source for the transmission of organisms, both macro- and microscopic, toxins, irritants and allergens. Maintaining nail cleanliness is essential to many aspects of health. The nail is also a focus of great importance; for many, cleanliness alone does not achieve aesthetic satisfaction. A multitude of products, implements and procedures are now on sale to enhance the appearance of nails (and, therefore, fingertips). While the cosmetic industry encourages and caters for the trappings of nail care and adornment, the motivation is probably innate; nail beautification was an established practice in societies long past; the long fingernail, often accentuated by gold and jewelled fingertip extenders, was indicative of high rank and station in society. Thus for social, cosmetic and cultural reasons and to aid normal function of digits with abnormal nails it is important to consider cosmetic, podiatric or chiropody treatment for dystrophies in which cure is not possible.

There are a great many nail conditions which need camouflage. Several factors should be taken into account:

- Age of patient
- Sex
- Type and origin of the dystrophy
- Affected part of the nail apparatus: nail plate or distal phalanx

Brittle nails

Nail brittleness causes several clinical symptoms including splitting, softening, lamellar exfoliation and onychorrhexis. Brittle nails are a common complaint. They are often an idiopathic condition, but can also be a symptom of a large number of dermatological nail disorders. Although brittle nails have been linked with many internal diseases, the high frequency of nail fragility in the general population makes it difficult to prove the validity of any such association. Environmental and occupational factors that produce a progressive dehydration of the nail plate play an important role in the development of idiopathic nail brittleness. Management of brittle nails requires preventive and protective measures to avoid nail plate dehydration. Affected individuals should wear cotton gloves under rubber gloves during household tasks, avoid repeated immersion in soap and water and keep their nails short. Nail varnishes may be protective, but the use of nail varnish remover should be limited since it exacerbates brittleness.

Local therapies are useful in the treatment of nail brittleness. Application of hydrophilic petrolatum on wet nails at bed time helps to retain the moisture in the nail plate. Frequent application of topical preparations containing hydrophilic substances such as phospholipids, hyaluronic acid, α-hydroxy acids and proteoglycans may favour nail plate rehydration.

Nail wrapping limited to the distal portion of the nail may afford protection and camouflage in recalcitrant fragility of the nail keratin. Oral treatment with biotin 2.5 mg per day for several months and even all year round can be useful as it may improve the synthesis of the lipid molecules that produce binding between nail plate corneocytes.

Cosmetic treatment of nail dystrophies

Cosmetics available for this purpose include:

- Nail varnish; stick-on nail dressing
- Preformed artificial nail
- Sculptured artificial nail
- Nail wrapping
- Adaptable nail prosthesis
- Abrader

Nail varnish

Nail varnish may hide any type of chromonychia in women (even very young) if the surface of the nail plate is smooth, or if it can be rendered so by fine sandpaper.

The hue resulting from *Pseudomonas* nail infection is often hidden by nail varnish, which may be kept on during the treatment with chlorox and is a helpful therapy for this condition. Psoriasis may benefit from the use of nail varnish under some circumstances.

Stick-on nail dressing ('Press-on' nail polish)

This consists of a very thin coloured synthetic film with an adhesive which fixes it firmly to the nail.

The changes produced on the nail vary considerably in intensity from patient to patient: flaking, roughness, ridging, onycholysis, disappearance of the lunula and disorganization of the nail plate which may be delaminated and broken off can be observed; mild paronychial inflammation with loss of the cuticle may be seen.

In some instances 9 or 12 months will pass before the nails have entirely returned to normal. The effect on the nail is simply traumatic, not allergic, a combination of the impermeability of the adhering film and the cumulative trauma to the nail plate when the film is repeatedly pulled off.

Preformed artificial nail

Any dystrophy may be corrected by preformed artificial nails, providing that some natural nail plate surface is still present to allow adequate adhesion. It is obvious that a severe dystrophy will prevent this and the usefulness of such a prosthetic nail is then limited. Local complications may appear when preformed artificial nails remain on for 3 or 4 days.

Distant allergic eczematous contact dermatitis may occur, more often due to the glue than to the prosthetic nail itself.

Sculptured artificial nails

Some natural nail keratin must be present for sculptured artificial nails to be used. The natural nail is first roughened with a burr, then painted with the acrylic resins which harden at room temperature and become moulded on to the nail. The prosthesis can be filed and manicured to shape. As the nail grows out, further applications of the self-curing acrylic resins can be made to maintain a regular contour.

Allergic contact dermatitis may appear, generally after 2 to 4 months of application, as distant sensitization (face, eyelids) or local reactions (onychial and paronychial tissues). On patch testing, the patient may react strongly to the acrylic liquid monomer.

Nail wrapping

Essentially, the free edge of each nail is splinted with layers of a fibrous substance such as cotton wool, paper or plastic film and affixed with a variety of glues; after drying, the edge is fashioned to requirements and the nail is coated with enamel. The entire procedure is repeated every 2 weeks. Nail wrapping is useful but can do significant harm if the entire nail is covered because of the occlusive nature of the material used. Allergic reactions to cyanoacrylate nail preparations (painful paronychia, onychodystrophy, discoloration and even exceptional permanent nail loss) are rare, but may persist for more than a year.

Adaptable nail prosthesis

In a wide variety of cases, ranging from deformed nails to complete loss of the distal phalanx, and in women particularly, a silicone rubber thimble-shaped finger cover may be employed. The fixation is excellent. The device is easy to clean (plain soap), flame-resistant, and the formed nail takes varnish well.

Nail abrasion

Thick nails caused by diseases such as psoriasis, pityriasis rubra pilaris and pachyonychia congenita can be abraded. Hyperkeratosis is prone to be associated with onychomycosis of the toes. Nail abrasion helps to expose the nail bed to anti-fungal chemicals, especially in the elderly where systemic treatment is not advisable. Abrasion is a good way to improve the contour of an abnormal nail, for example in onychogryphosis.

In selected cases of ingrowing toe nail, repeated thinning of the nail plate may be a useful conservative method in association with appropriate definitive treatment. There are many products, implements and devices for maintaining clean, well groomed nails to satisfy individual needs. These benefits are obtained with small risk. The physician can and should be well versed in nail care and adornment to aid patients in achieving an improved, positive self-image: when specific medical cure is shown to be impossible, the physician will then be in a good position to judge the value of cosmetic, chiropody or podiatry treatments.

Acute paronychia

Acute paronychia is usually caused by *Staphylococcus aureus*, although other bacteria and herpes simplex may occasionally be responsible. Minor trauma commonly precedes the infection. Whenever possible cultures should be taken.

Treatment includes local treatment with antiseptics (chlorhexidine, betadine) and administration of systemic antibiotics. If acute paronychia does not show clear signs of response to penicillinase-resistant antibiotics within two days, then surgical treatment should be instituted using proximal block anaesthesia. The base of the nail is removed by cutting across with pointed scissors.

Blistering distal dactylitis

This is a childhood disease usually caused by *S. aureus*, characterized by bullous lesions with purulent content localized at the tip of the digits. Treatment includes surgical drainage of the blisters, topical medication with antiseptics and systemic antibiotics (oral erythromycin or amoxycillin).

Chronic paronychia

Chronic paronychia represents an inflammatory reaction of the proximal nail fold to irritants or allergens. It affects hands that are continually exposed to a wet environment and to multiple microtrauma, favouring cuticle damage. Secondary colonization with *Candida albicans* and/or bacteria occurs in most cases. Patients with chronic paronychia should avoid a wet environment, chronic microtrauma and contact with irritants or allergens.

High-potency topical steroids (clobetasol propionate 0.05%) once a day at bed time are an effective first line therapy. If *Candida* is present a topical imidazole derivative should be applied in the morning. Topical anti-fungals alone and systemic anti-fungals are not useful. In severe cases, intralesional or even systemic steroids (prednisone 20

mg/day) can be used for a few days to obtain a prompt reduction of inflammation and pain. Acute exacerbations of chronic paronychia do not necessitate antibiotic treatment since they subside spontaneously in a few days. *Pseudomonas* colonization can be treated with sodium hypochlorite solution or 2% acetic acid. Complete recovery of the condition usually requires several weeks and treatment should be continued until the cuticle has regrown. Recurrences are frequent since the barrier function of the proximal nail fold may be impaired for months or even years after an episode of chronic paronychia. In rare cases, foreign bodies such as hair or fibre glass spicules can be responsible for chronic paronychia. These patients should be treated by the excision of a crescent shaped, full thickness piece of the proximal nail fold, including its swollen portion. Complete healing by granulation takes about 4 weeks.

Onycholysis

Onycholysis describes the detachment of the nail plate from the nail bed. Starting from the central or lateral portion of the nail plate free margin, onycholysis progresses proximally and can even involve the whole nail. The onycholytic area looks whitish because of the presence of air under the detached nail plate. It may occasionally show a greenish or brown discoloration due to colonization of the onycholytic space by chromogenic bacteria (*Pseudomonas aeruginosa*), moulds or yeasts. Onycholysis may be idiopathic or represent a symptom of numerous diseases such as psoriasis, onychomycosis, contact dermatitis or drug reactions. Depending on the cause of the complaint (e.g. onychomycosis, psoriasis, impaired peripheral circulation), appropriate local treatment, systemic treatment or both is prescribed.

The detached nail should be clipped away and a mild antibacterial solution (thymol 4% in chloroform) should be applied on the exposed nail bed at night. Pseudomonas infection is easily treated by using sodium hypochlorite solution or 2% acetic acid. Accurate drying of the fingers after hand washing is necessary. A hair dryer may be useful for this purpose.

Psoriasis

Since treatment of nail psoriasis is always disappointing, before treatment is started the individual problems of every patient should be carefully considered, and in particular the degree of discomfort that results from the nail lesions. Reassuring the patient is probably the best approach for isolated nail pitting, oily patches, mild onycholysis and splinter haemorrhages. However, diffuse onycholysis, subungual hyperkeratosis and severe nail plate surface abnormalities may require a positive therapeutic approach.

Local therapies of nail psoriasis are scarcely effective and only rarely induce complete remission of the disease. Topical steroids or combinations of topical steroids with salicylic acid and/or retinoic acid are widely prescribed. Their efficacy is poor, even when applied with occlusive dressing after chemical or mechanical avulsion of the onycholytic nail plate. Long-term application of topical steroids may result in marked atrophy of the soft tissues of the digits or even in focal resorption of the distal phalanges. Topical calcipotriol may be effective when onycholysis and subungual hyperkeratosis are prominent symptoms.

In patients with pustular psoriasis local treatment with topical anti-metabolites (mechlorethamine, 1% fluorouracil) is an option, even though results are variable. Possible side-effects limit the utilization of these drugs in uncomplicated nail psoriasis.

Topical psoralens followed by UVA exposure are scarcely effective due to poor penetration of the UVA through the nail plate, especially when thickened. However, topical PUVA may be useful in pustular psoriasis when recurrent pustular lesions have produced destruction of the nail plate. Intralesional injections of triamcinolone acetonide 10 mg/ml, at a dose of 0.2 to 0.5 ml per nail, have been proven effective in some cases of nail matrix psoriasis.

In patients with nail plate surface abnormalities the steroids should be injected in the nail matrix, whereas in patients with subungual hyperkeratosis the site of injection should be the nail bed. Injections should be repeated monthly for 6 months, then every 6 weeks for the next 6 months and finally every 2 months for 6 to 12 months. A digital block is sometimes useful to make the treatment less painful, but when several digits are involved, a wrist block may be the appropriate anaesthesia. However, routine use of this treatment is not recommended due to the pain caused by the injections, the local side-effects and relapses of the nail abnormalities after discontinuation of the therapy.

Systemic treatment with methotrexate or cyclosporin A can clear the nail changes, but this can be recommended only when nail psoriasis is associated with widespread disease or psoriatic arthritis.

Retinoids are only of little value in the treatment of nail psoriasis except for hyperkeratotic nails. Oral administration of etretinate or acitretin can even worsen the nail changes due to the development of nail brittleness, pyogenic granuloma-like lesions and chronic paronychia. Oral photochemotherapy can improve crumbling of the nail plate and psoriatic involvement of the proximal nail fold, but is scarcely effective in nail pitting or in subungual hyperkeratosis. Superficial radiotherapy can have a beneficial effect on psoriatic nails but is not recommended due to its short-term benefits.

. Pustular psoriasis of the nail unit usually fails to respond to conventional topical treatments. Retinoids, systemic steroids, PUVA and cyclosporin can arrest the development of pustular lesions and avoid permanent scarring of the nail apparatus.

Lichen planus

Specific nail involvement occurs in about 10% of patients with lichen planus and permanent damage of at least one nail occurs in approximately 4% of patients. However, if lichen planus is correctly diagnosed and treated, permanent damage to the nail unit is rare, even in patients with diffuse involvement of the nail matrix.

Systemic steroids are effective in treating nail lichen planus. Oral prednisone 0.5 mg/ kg every other day for 2 to 6 weeks or intramuscular triamcinolone acetonide 0.5 mg/kg every month for 2 to 3 months usually produces recovery of the nail abnormalities. Intralesional injections of triamcinolone acetonide 10 mg/ml represent a possible, but painful, alternative when the disease is limited to a few finger nails. Mild relapses are frequently observed, but recurrences are usually responsive to therapy.

Systemic retinoids at dosages utilized for psoriasis are a good alternative.

Twenty nail dystrophy

This condition, characterized by nail roughness, can be idiopathic or associated with alopecia areata and less often with lichen planus. It is a benign condition that never causes nail scarring. The nail changes usually regress spontaneously in a few years. Reassuring the patient is probably the best approach for this nail disorder. Although

topical PUVA can be effective, continuous treatment is required to maintain the results.

Yellow nail syndrome

This is an uncommon disorder of unknown aetiology, characterized by the triad of yellow nails, lymphoedema and respiratory tract involvement.

Vitamin E at dosages ranging from 600 to 1200 IU daily can induce a complete clearing of the nail changes. Although the mechanism of action of vitamin E in yellow nail syndrome is still unknown, antioxidant properties of α-tocopherol may account for its efficacy. A 5% solution of vitamin E in dimethyl sulphoxide produced marked clinical improvement in a double-blind controlled study. The efficacy of topical vitamin E, however, still needs confirmation.

Oral itraconazole, 400 mg daily one week a month for several months, may be beneficial.

Onychogryphosis

Chemical avulsion of the overgrowing nail plate with urea ointment is useful and provides considerable relief of the patient's discomfort. Different formulations can be used, ranging from a simple 40% urea in 60% white petrolatum preparation to the the South & Farber ointment that has the following formulation:

Urea 40%
White beeswax 5%
Anhydrous lanolin 20%
White petrolatum 25%
Micronized silica gel 10%

Before the ointment is applied on the nail plate surface, it is mandatory to cover the periungual skin with plastic tape in order to protect the skin from maceration. The urea ointment is then applied on the nail and covered with a plastic wrap; the medication is fixed to the digit with a plastic tape and maintained in place for 7 to 10 days. Finally, the medication is wiped off and the softened nail plate is removed using nail clippers.

Chemical nail avulsion is only effective when the nail plate is partially or totally detached from the nail bed. It is not useful on normal nails, but can be successfully utilized to remove onychomycotic nails as well as thickened psoriatic nails.

Nail biting and onychotillomania

Frequent application of distasteful topical preparations on the nail and periungual skin can discourage patients from biting and chewing their fingernails. Possible alternatives include:

- 1% Clindamycin
- Quaternary ammonium derivatives
- 4% Quinine sulphate in petrolatum

Patients with severe onychophagia or median nail dystrophy can be helped by daily bandaging the injured fingers with micropore.

Periungual warts

Periungual and subungual warts are usually difficult to treat and frequently recur. The lifespan of periungual warts may be such that they, and the various treatments, may exceed the patience of both patient and physician! Under such circumstances intelli-

gent placebo therapy may well be appropriate. A great variety of treatments are listed in all pharmacopoeias, reflecting their individually limited success rates.

> **Procrastination may sometimes be the best treatment for periungual warts**

Topical immunotherapy

Topical immunotherapy with strong topical sensitizers (squaric acid dibutylester (SADBE), diphenylcyclopropenone) is an effective and painless modality of treatment for multiple warts. SADBE or diphenylcyclopropenone 2% in acetone is used for sensitization. After 21 days, weekly applications are carried out with dilutions from 0.001% to 1% according to the patient's response. Complete cure usually requires 3 to 4 months.

Cimetidine

Multiple warts can also be treated with cimetidine 750–1200 mg daily for 3 to 4 months. The efficacy of the drug is possibly related to its immunomodulatory effects.

Cantharidin

Cantharone Plus (30% salicylic acid, 5% podophyllin, 1% cantharidin) is designed for topical application to the wart and within a 1 to 3 mm margin around the wart by the physician in the office; occasionally the nail must be trimmed to expose subungual warts to the medication. When dry the wart is covered by a piece of Blenderm (a topical steroid in a transparent adhesive film). The resultant blister is painful and inflamed. The next day the wart tissue is treated by curettage under local anaesthesia. This treatment is not recommended for use in young children due to difficulties in pain management.

Liquid nitrogen

The use of liquid nitrogen is convenient and efficient, but lesions frozen around the nails may produce throbbing, intense pain, secondary to oedema under the nail bed. One must also be aware that the skin of both infants and the elderly often swells more than might normally be expected in inter-mediate age groups.

Haemorrhagic bullae may be cosmetically unpleasant but usually painless: they develop within 12 to 24 hours and remain for about 7 to 10 days before drying. Their premature rupture does not alter the course of healing.

Application of clobetasol propionate, under occlusion, before treatment reduces the inflammatory response to the freeze and may be continued twice a day for 2 to 3 days. Oral aspirin 500 mg, three times daily, commenc-ing 2 hours before and for 3 days after treat-ment minimizes pain.

Bleomycin

Intralesional injections of bleomycin have been successfully used to treat viral warts for many years. The powder should be diluted to a concentration of 1 unit per ml with saline. This solution can be stored at $-20°C$ in glass for several months. Part of this solution should be further diluted to 0.1–0.5 units per ml and injected into multiple loci of the warts. Patients with vascular impairment and women of child-bearing age should not

be treated because the drug has been reported to produce Raynaud's disease and to be systemically absorbed.

We advise Shelley and Shelley's technique: a bifurcate vaccination needle introduces bleomycin (1 unit per ml sterile saline solution) into warts using multiple punctures. After local anaesthesia the bleomycin solution is dropped onto the wart, which is then punctured with a disposable bifurcated needle approximately 40 times per 5 mm^2 area of the wart. No medications are required. Three weeks after treatment, the eschar can be pared away and the area examined for residual warts, which can be retreated. This technique minimizes the amount of bleomycin introduced into the skin.

Electrodesiccation

Electrodesiccation can produce unsightly scarring. Removal of subungual and periun-gual warts by blunt dissection offers a surgi-cal alternative when conventional measures fail.

Carbon dioxide laser

On fingers the warts must be followed down fully into the sulcus of the lateral nail fold. Using a minimally defocused beam of less than 1 mm spot size allows the complete tracing out of the tumour. For subungual warts the laser should be used to ablate 'interfering' portions of nail plate and the wart can easily be vaporized subsequently. Complications such as permanent nail dystrophy after ablation of periungual warts are rarely observed.

Index

Page numbers in *italic* refer to the illustrations

Abrasion, 201
Abscesses, 91–2, 194
Acetic acid, 202, 203
Acidophilic masses, 4
Acitretin, 203
Acquired periungual fibrokeratoma, 99, 101, 103–5, *105*
Acral lentiginous melanoma, 116, 120
Acro-osteolysis, 23, 194
Acrocephalosyndactyly, 34
Acrochordon, 105
Acrodermatitis, *94*
Acrodermatitis continua, 126
Acrodermatitis enteropathica, 58, 72, 93
Acrodysostosis, 34
Acrokeratosis paraneoplastica, 78, 121, 130–1, *130*
Acrokeratosis verruciformis, 146
Acromegaly, 20, 21, *22*, 23, 26
Acropustuloses, 121, 126–7, *127*, *128*
Acrosclerosis, 42, *45*, 86
Acrylic sculptured nails, *181*, 182
Actidione, 163
Actinic keratosis, 101
Actinic reticuloid, 70
Acute paronychia, 89–91, *90*, 126, 171, 194, *195*, *196*, 201–2

Acyclovir, 123, 147
Adaptable nail prostheses, 201
Addison's disease, 116, 147
Adrenal insufficiency, 100
Adriamycin, 147
AIDS, 21, 114, 118, 146, 151, 157
Albumin, 143
Alcohol, 23, 39
Alimentary tract disorders, 23
Alkaline metabolic disease, 146
Alopecia areata, 26, 54, 59, 60–1, *60*, *61*, 63, 70, 78, 137, 144, 146, *153*
Alopecia totalis, 60–1
Alopecia unguium, 72
α–hydroxy acids, 200
Alteration of nail, *187–90*, 188–90
Amelogenesis imperfecta, 72
Amoebiasis, 23
Amorolfine, 165
Amoxycillin, 202
Amyloidosis, 42, 63, 83, 100, *135*, 137, 147
Anaemia, 60, 70, 83, 137, 139, 144, 146, 151
Anatomy, 1–4, *2*
Aneurysmal bone cyst, 101, 194
Aneurysms, 21, 23, 76
Angiokeratoma, 100
Angiokeratoma circumscriptum, 101
Angioma, 101, 151
Anonychia, 42, *43*, *44*, 189

Antibiotics, 72, 89, 202
Antifungals, 165, 201, 202
Antimalarial drugs, 100, 151, *152*
Antimetabolite drugs, 137, 203
Antimony poisoning, 146
Antimycotics, 165
Antiphospholipid syndrome, 83
Antiseptics, 202
Aortic aneurysm, 21, 23
Aplastic anonychia, 42, 72
Apparent leukonychia, 140, 142–4, *143*, *145*
Argyria, 151
Arsenic, 23, 100, 137, 146
Arsenic keratosis, 78, 101
Arterial emboli, 83
Arterial graft sepsis, 19, 21, 23
Arteries, 4, *5*
Arteriovenous fistula, 101
Arteriovenous shunts, 7
Arthritis, 83, 107, 110, 133, 195
Arthropathy, 137
Artificial nails, 200–1
Ascariasis, 23
Aspergillus, 151
Aspirin, 176, 206
Asthma, 21
Atopic dermatitis, 39, 60, 70
Atypical melanocytic hyperplasia, 101
Aureomycin, 124
Autoimmune thrombocytopenic purpura, 60
Ayerza's syndrome, 21
AZT, 116

Bacteria, paronychia, 90, 91–2, 201
Basal cell carcinoma, 100, 101, 147
Bazex's acrokeratosis paraneoplastica, 78
Beau's lines, 6, 7, 55–8, *55–7*, 59, 71–2, 171
Behçet's disease, 83
Benign juvenile digital fibromatosis, 101, 106, *106*
Benign melanocytic hyperplasia, 101
Berk–Tabatznik syndrome, 34
Beryllium poisoning, 23
Betadine, 202
Bifid toe, 39, *41*
Bifonazole, 165
Biopsy, malignant melanoma, 120
Biotin, 200
Biting nails, 33, *33*, 47, 92, 93–6, 189, 205
Black nails, 147–9, *148–51*
'Black superficial onychomycosis', 158, 167
Blastomycosis, 21
Blenderm, 205
Bleomycin, *57*, 70, 101, 151, 206
Blistering distal dactylitis (BDD), 121, 124–5, *125*, 202
Blood dyscrasias, 83, 84
Blood supply, 4, *5*, 6–7
Blue nails, 151
Bone, subungual exostosis, 108, *109*, *174*, 191
Bourneville–Pringle disease, 38, 99, 103
Bowen's disease, 78, 99, 100, 101, 112–13, *112*, *113*, 114, 117, 118, 147, 194
Brachial artery cannula, 83
Brachial plexus injury, 21
Brachydactylia, 33
Brachyonychia, *31–3*, 33–4, *35*, 36
Breast carcinoma, 147
Brittle nails, 133–7, 189, 199–200
Bronchiectasis, 21
Broncho–pulmonary disease, 21
Brown nails, 147–9, *148–51*
Buerger's disease, 83
Bulla repens, 89

Bullous diseases, 70, 72, 85, 87, 151
Bullous ichthyosiform, 7
Bullous impetigo, 124, 125
Bunell's technique, paronychia, 89–90
Burns, 87, 125
Butcher's nodule, 99–100

Cachexic states, 133, 137
Calcipotriol, 203
Calcium, 4, 136
Calluses, 35, 177
Candida, 71, 91, 92, 125–6, *166*, 167–8, 202
Cantharidin, 100, 205–6
Cantharone Plus, 205
Captopril, 70
Carbon dioxide laser treatment, 206
Carbon monoxide poisoning, 139
Carcinoma:
  alimentary tract, 23
  basal cell, 100, 101, 147
  breast, 147
  epidermoid, 112–13, *112*, *113*, *196*
  lung, 18, 19, 70, 146
  squamous cell, 99, 100, 101, 113–14, 194
Cardiac failure, 151
Cardiovascular disease, 21–3
Carotene, 151
Carpal tunnel syndrome, 26, 56, 147
Castellani's paint, *150*
Causalgia, 107
Cautery, hot paper clip, 83
Cell kinetics, 5–6
Cephalexin, 124
Cephaloridine, 70
Chemicals, fragile nails, 137
Chemotherapy, *55*, 116, 128, 143, 146
Chilblains, 194
Childhood, 6
Chloramphenicol, 70, 163
Chlorohexidine, 202
Chlorpromazine, 70, 147
Chondrodysplasia punctata, 65
Chromogenic bacteria, 100
Chromonychia, 139–53, *140–53*, 200
Chromosomal abnormalities, 39

Chronic paronychia, 21, 91–3, *93*, 125–6, *126*, 194, 202
Cicatricial pemphigoid, 42, 87
Ciclopirox, 165
Cimetidine, 205
Cirrhosis, 23, 83, 84, 142, 146
Cirsoid tumours, 54, 151
Clavus, subungual, 177
Claw-like nails, 35–7, *37*
Claw toes, 176
Clindamycin, 205
Clioquinole, 151
Clobetasol propionate, 202, 206
Cloxacillin, 70
Clubbing, 17–23, *17*, *18*, *20*, *22*, *32*
Coffin–Siris syndrome, 42
COIF syndrome, *38*
Cold injury, 194
Collagen, 4
Collagen vascular disease, 54, 83, 84, 93
'Collar–stud' abscesses, 91
Colonic diseases, 23
Colour changes, 139–53, *140–53*
Coloured lines, 54
Connective tissue, 4
Consistency, nail, 133–7, *133–6*
Contact dermatitis, 70, 78, 91, 93, 200, 201
Convoluted nail, 183
Copper staining, *151*
Corneocytes, 7
Corns, subungual, 99, 101, 177, *177*, *178*, 194
Corticosteroids, 111
Cortisone, 146
Cosmetic treatments, nail dystrophies, 200–1
Cryoglobulinaemia, 83, 84
Cryosurgery, 101–2, 111, 194
Cryptogenic hyperkeratosis, *75*
Cushing's disease, 100, 147
Cutaneous horn, 105
Cuticle, 2, 3
  biting and picking, 187
  nervous habits, 57
  ragged, 93–6, *97*
  removal, 137
Cyanoacrylate nail preparations, 201
Cyanosis, 21
Cycloheximide, 163, 167

Cyclophosphamide, 147
Cyclosporin, 203, 204
Cystine, 136
Cysts:
    aneurysmal bone cysts, 101, 194
    epidermal cysts, 100, 101, 194
    implantation cysts, *197*
    myxoid cysts, 50, *53*, 99, 101, 108–12, *110, 111*, 191, *191*, 194
Cytotoxic drugs, *55, 56,* 58, 72, 100, 146, 147

Darier's disease:
    brittle nails, *136,* 137
    koilonychia, 26
    leukonychia, 144, 146
    linear red line, 151
    longitudinal grooves, 50, 54
    paronychia, 93
    splinter haemorrhages, 83
    thick nails, 72, 78, *80*
    worn down nails, *41,* 42
Demethylchlortetracycline, 70
Dermatitis, 39, 60, 70, 91, 93, 146, 200, 201
Dermatofibroma, 101, 103
Dermatofibrosarcoma, 105
Dermatomyositis, 93, 97
Dermatophytes, onychomycosis, 151, 155–65, *155–64*
Dermis, 3
Diabetes, 10, 92
Diamond's syndrome, 23
Digital arteries, 4, *5*
Digital nerves, 4, *5*
Dimethylsulphoxide (DMSO), 163
Diphencyprone, 100, 205
Diphenylcyclopropenone, 100, 205
Distal joint alteration, 191
Distal nail embedding, 179–82, *180–6*
Distal subungual onychomycosis (DSO), 155–7, *155–8,* 162, *162,* 167
Dithranol, 147
Diuretics, 70
DNA, 5
Dolichonychia, 30, *31*
DOOR syndrome, 42, *43*

Dorsal pterygium, 84–6, *85, 86,* 87
Dorsolateral fissures, 96–8, *98,* 194
Doxorubicin, 70
Doxycycline, 70
Drugs:
    addiction, 23
    antifungals, 165
    benign lesions, 100
    brittle nails, 137
    leukonychia, 146
    longitudinal melanonychia, 114, 116
    melanonychia, 147
    nail shedding, 72
    onycholysis, 70
    splinter haemorrhages, 83, 84
    yellow nails, 151
Dwarfism, nanocephalic, 34
Dyshidrosis, 144, 146
Dyskeratosis congenita, 39, 87, 93, 136
Dysmenorrhoea, 56, 58
Dystrophia longitudinalis fissuriformis, 50–1

Eccrine poroma, 105
Eccrine sweat glands, 4
Ectodermal dysplasia, *25, 26, 39,* 39, *43, 44,* 63
Ectrodactyly, 42
Eczema:
    fragile nails, 137
    paronychia, 91, 92, 93
    pitting, 59, 60
    splinter haemorrhages, 83
    thick nails, 78
    trachyonychia, 61, 63
    transverse lines, 56, 58
    worn down nails, 42
'Egg-shell nails', 135
Ehlers Danlos syndrome, 30
Eikenella corrodens, 126
Electrodesiccation, warts, 206
Elephantiasis, 76
Emboli, 83, 84
Emetine, 146
Emphysema, 21
Encephalitis, 93
Enchondroma, 99, 101, 151, 194
Endocarditis, bacterial, 84
Endocrine disorders, 23, 70, 114, 116

Endonyx onychomycosis (EO), 155, 158–62, *161*
Epidermal cysts, 100, 101, 194
Epidermal naevi, 101
Epidermis, 3, 6
Epidermoid carcinoma, 99, 112–13, *112, 113, 196*
Epidermolysis bullosa, 42, *45,* 125
Epiloia, 38, 103, 104
Epoxy resin dermatitis, 93
Erosions, 58
Erythema multiforme, 146
Erythroderma, 7, 39, 78
Erythromelalgia, 23
Erythromycin, 124, 125, 202
Etretinate, 42, *44, 94,* 137, 203
Eunuchoidism, 30
Exfoliative dermatitis, 146
Exostosis, 105, 194
    hereditary multiple, 101
    subungual, 100, 101, 108, *109,* 172, *174*

Familial mandibuloacral dysplasia, 34
Familial polyposis, 23
Fasting, 146
Fat cells, 3–4
Fetal hydantoin syndrome, 147
Fever:
    nail shedding, 72
    transverse grooves, 58
Fibrokeratoma, 103–5, *105*
Fibromas, 101, 102–6, *103,* 194
Fibrosarcoma, 105
Finger tip, painful fissures, 96–8, *98,* 194
Fissures:
    dorsolateral, 96–8, *98,* 194
    nail, *133,* 172, *172*
    see also Splitting
Fluconazole, 165
Flumequine, 70
Fluoride poisoning, 146
Fluorouracil, 70, 203
Foot:
    gait cycle, 8, 9–10
    and toe nail problems, 7–15
    shape, 10
Footwear *see* Shoes
Foreign bodies, 93, 100, 194, 202
Formaldehyde nail hardeners, 87
Formalin, 102

Fractures, 146
Fragile nails, 133–7, *134*, *135*, 199–200
Frictional melanonychia, 115, 189–90, *190*
Frostbite, 54, 93
Fuchsin nail staining, *150*
Fungal infections:
  brittle nails, 136
  melanonychia, 114, 147
  onychomycosis, 155–68, *155–66*
Fusarium, 167
Fusarium oxysporum, 92

Gait cycle, positions of foot, 8, 9–10
Gardner's syndrome, 23
Garlic clove fibroma, 103, *105*
Germinative matrix, 3
Giant cell tumour, 101
Glomus tumour, 4, *53*, 54, 99, 101, 106–8, *107*, 151, 193, 194, *197*
Glycoprotein, 69
Gold salts, 137
Gonorrhoea, 121, 123
Gout, 21, 23, 107, 137, 146, 194
Graft-versus-host disease, 42, 87, 137
Gram-negative enteric bacteria, 90
Granuloma, foreign body, 93, 100
Green nails, 151
Griseofulvin, 165
Grooves, longitudinal, 49–52, *49–53*
Growth of nails, 5–7

Haemangioendothelioma, 100
Haematoma, subungual, 82–4, 149, *149*, 151, *195*
  differential diagnosis of malignant melanoma, 100, 119–20
  trauma, 10, 169–71, *169*, *170*, *175*, 176, *176*
  treatment, 83, 84
  vitamin C deficiency, *82*
Haemochromatosis, 26, 83, 147
Haemodialysis, 83, 137
Haemoglobinopathies, 23
Haemorrhage:

melanonychia, 147
  splinter haemorrhages, 80–3, *81*, *82*, 84, 170
Hailey–Hailey disease, 144, *145*
Half-and-half nail of Lindsay, 144, *144*, 146
Hallopeau's acrodermatitis, 93, 115, 126, *127*
Hallux nail pathology, 174
Hallux rigidus, 10
Hallux valgus, *9*, 10, 76, 174, *175*
Hammer toes, 176, 177
Hand–foot–mouth disease, 121
Haneke's technique, pincer nail, 185, *185*
Hang nail, 93–6, *98*, 187
Hapalonychia, 133–7
Hashish, 21, 23
Heart disease, 21–3, 83, *153*
Heel height, shoes, 11–12
Heller's median canaliform dystrophy, 52, *52*, 54, 188
Heloma, *177*, *178*
Hemiplegia, 133, 137
Hendersonula toruloidea, 116, 167
Henna, *150*
Heparin, 151
Hepatitis, 23
Hereditary multiple exostosis, 101
Heroin, 21, 23
Herpes simplex, 70, 91, 121–3, *122*, 126, 194, *195*, 201
Herpes zoster, 70, 123, *197*
Herringbone nails, 53, *54*
Hidrotic ectodermal dysplasia, 27, *40*
High altitudes purpura, 83
Hippocrates, 17
Hippocratic fingers, 17–23
Histiocytosis-X, 83, 84, 93
HIV, 116, 157
Hjorth–Sabouraud syndrome, 92, 128–30, *129*
Hodgkin's disease, 21, 146
Hook nail, 21, *22*, 35, 37, *37*, 172
HPV virus, 114
Hutchinson's sign, 117–18, 120
Hyaluronic acid, 200
Hydantoinates, 39
Hydrophilic petrolatum, 200
Hydroxyapatite crystals, 4

Hyperhidrosis, 70
Hyperkeratosis, 72–80, *75–80*
  causes, 75, 76
  claw–like nails, 35
  onychomycosis, 156, *156*, *157*, 201
  parakeratosis pustulosa, 129
  thick nails, 78
  trauma, 173, *173*, 176–8, 179, *179*
Hyperostosis, *179*
Hyperparathyroidism, 33, *35*
Hyperpigmentation, *115*, 117
Hypertension, 83
Hyperthyroidism, 7, 137
Hypertrophic pulmonary osteoarthropathy, 19, 20
Hypertrophic scars, 102
Hypertrophy, 72–80, *75–80*
Hypertrophy of the lateral lip, 186–7, *186*
Hyperuricaemia, 76
Hypervitaminosis A, 23
Hypoalbuminaemia, 143, *143*, 146
Hypocalcaemia, 146
Hypohidrotic ectodermal dysplasia, 27, 30
Hyponychium, 3, 72
Hypoparathyroidism, 58, 72, 83
Hypopituitarism, 30
Hypothyroidism, 7, 70, 133, 137
Hypoxia, 23

Ichthyosis, 72, 76, 78
Ichthyosis vulgaris, 60, 63
Idiopathic atrophy of childhood, 42
Idiopathic onycholysis of women, 7
Idiopathic trachyonychia, 60, 61, *62*, 63
IgA deficiency, 60, 63
Imidazole, 167, 202
Immunotherapy, warts, 205
Impetigo, 89, 121, 124, *124*, 125
Implantation cyst, *197*
Incontinentia pigmenti, 101, 194
Infants:
  Beau's lines, 56
  koilonychia, 25, *25*
  Veillonella infection, 123–4

Infections, acute paronychia, 89–91
Inflammation:
  longitudinal melanonychia, 114, 115–16
  paronychia, 93–6
Inflammatory bowel disease, 21
Ingrowing nails, 10, 91, 93, 100, 121, 173, 179–82, *180–6*, 194, *197*, 201
Insecticides, 27, *29*
Iron deficiency, 25, 26, 70, 136, 137
Irradiation, 114, 147
Ischaemia, 91, 93, 133, 194
Iso Kikuchi syndrome, 37–8
Isolated longitudinal leukonychia, 142
Isotretinoin, *94*
Itraconazole, 165, 168, 204

Jaundice, 151
Jogger's toe, 176
Joints, alteration, 191
Junctional naevi, 100, 116
Juvenile ingrowing toenail, 185–6, *186*

Kaposi's sarcoma, 100, 101
Kawasaki syndrome, 58, 72
Keipert syndrome, 34
Keloids, 101, 102, 105
Keratin, 136, 140
Keratinization, 6
Keratinocytes, 3, 7
Keratoacanthoma, 99, 100, 101, 194
Keratohyalin, 3
Keratosis cristarum, 80
Keratosis punctata, 72
Ketoconazole, 147, 165, 168
Kidney transplants, 146
Knuckle pads, 60, 63
Koenen's tumour, 101, 103, *104*, 105
KOH preparations, 162–3, *163*
Koilonychia, 6, 23–6, *24–6*, 61, *145*, 146, 189
Kwashiorkor, 7, 23

Lamellar splitting, 63–5, *63*, *64*, 135
Lamina, nail plate, 4
Langerhans cell histiocytosis, 84
Larsen's syndrome, 34

Laser treatment, 102, 206
Lateral nail folds, 1, 2
Laugier–Hunziker–Baran syndrome, 100, 101, 114, *115*, 118, 147
Lead poisoning, 146
Lectitis purulenta et granulomatosa, 69
Leiomyoma, 101, 194
Lentigines, 147
Lentigo–naevus, 118
Lentigo simplex, 101
LEOPARD syndrome, 26, 146
Leprosy, 133, 144, 146
Lesch–Nyhan syndrome, 42
Leukaemia, 93
Leuko-onycholysis paradentotica, 70, 146
Leukokoilonychia, *145*
Leukonychia, 25, 140–6, *140–5*, 190, *190*
Leukonychia variegata, 142
Lichen planus:
  dorsal pterygium, 84, *85*, 86, 87
  fragile nails, *134*, 137
  hyperkeratosis, 78, *80*
  koilonychia, 26
  longitudinal grooves, 49, *51*, 54
  melanonychia, 115, 147
  nail shedding, 72
  onychatrophy, 42, *46*
  onycholysis, 70
  onychoschizia, *64*, 65
  paronychia, 93
  pitting, 60
  red nails, 151
  trachyonychia, 61, *62*, 63
  treatment, 204
Lichen striatus, 52, 137
Linear nail growth, 6
Lines:
  longitudinal, 49–53, *49–53*, 54
  red, 151
  transverse, 53–8, *55–7*
Lipoma, 101
Liquid nitrogen, 206
Liver disease, 21
Long nails, 30, *31*
Longitudinal lines, 49–53, *49–53*, 54
Longitudinal melanonychia (LM), 100, 114–16, *114*, 147, *148*, 149, 171–2, 189, 190

Longitudinal ridges, 52–3
Lovibond, 19
Lung carcinoma, 18, 19, 70, 146
Lunula, 1, 3
  red, *153*
Lupus erythematosus, 23, 69, 70, 85, *95*, 151
Lyell syndrome, 42, 56, 72, *73*
Lymphangitis, 23
Lymphoma, 21, 42, 101

Macronychia, 37, 38, 39, *40*
Maffucci's syndrome, 23, 101
Malignant melanoma, 84, 101, 116–21, *117*, *119*, 147–9
Mallet toes, 176
Malnutrition, 21, 23, 118, 147
Manicures, onycholysis, 69, 71, *71*
Marfan's syndrome, 30, *31*
Measles, 56, 58
Mechlorethamine, 127, 203
Median canaliform dystrophy, 50–1, 52, *52*, 54, 58
Megadactyly, 38
Melanin, 84
Melanocytes, 3, 115–16
Melanocytic hyperplasia, 100, 116
Melanoma, 84, 99, 100, 101, 116–21, *117*, *119*, 147–9, 172
Melanonychia, 147–9, *148–51*, 189–90, *190*
Melanosomes, 115
Melanotic lesions, 101, 114–21, *114*, *115*, *117*, *119*
Menstrual cycle, 56, 58, 146
Mepacrine, 151
Mercury poisoning, 23
Mesothelioma, 19
Metastases, 21, 93, 99, 100, 101, 130, 194
Methaemoglobinaemia, 23
Methotrexate, 128, 203
Micronychia, 33, 37–8, *38–40*, 39, *43*
Microtrauma, 172–91, *175–91*
Minocycline, 70, 118, 151
Modifications of nail surface, 49–65, *49–64*
Monochloroacetic acid, 100
Muckle–Wells syndrome, 20
Mucoviscidosis, 21

Muehrcke's bands, 142, *143*, 146
Multicentric reticulohistiocytosis, 70, 101
Mycosis fungoides, 70
Myocardial infarction, 146
Myxoid pseudocysts, 50, *53*, 99, 101, 108–12, *110*, *111*, 191, *191*, 194
Myxoma, 23, 101

Naevi, 84, 100, 101, 116, 147, *148*
Naevocytic naevus, 101
Naevus flammeus, 101
Naevus striatus symmetricus, 51
Nail apparatus:
  blood supply, 4, *5*, 6–7
  in childhood, 6
  dynamics, 5–7
  microscopic anatomy, 3–4
  nerve supply, 4, *5*
  in old age, 6–7
  structure, 1–3, *2*
Nail artifacts, 189
Nail bed, anatomy, 1–2, 3–4
Nail biting, 33, *33*, 47, 92, 93–6, 189, 205
Nail braces, pincer nail, 183–5, *184*
Nail consistency, 133–7, *133–6*
Nail fold, 1, 2, 3
Nail matrix:
  microscopic anatomy, 3
  structure, 2–3
Nail matrix naevi, 116
Nail–patella syndrome, 26, 37, 39, 42, *44*, 52, 53, 54, *54*
Nail plate:
  abnormalities, 67–87, *67–86*
  anatomy, 4
  curvature, 4
  growth, 6
  hardness, 4
  structure, 1–2
Nail shedding, 71–2, *73*, *74*, 171, *188*, 189
Nail surface modifications, 49–65, *49–64*
Nail varnish, *134*, 136, 137, 140, 146, 151, 200
Nail wrapping, 52, 200, 201
Nanocephalic dwarfism, 34
'Neapolitan nails', 144

Neisseria gonorrhoeae, 123
Nerves, 4, *5*
Neuritis, 133
Neurodermatitis, 60
Neurogenic tumours, 101
Neuroma, 107, 194
Neuropathy, 137
Nitrogen, liquid, 206
Norwegian scabies, 78

Occupational problems:
  footwear, 15
  fragile nails, 133
  koilonychia, 25, 26
  pitting, 59, 60
  worn down nails, 42
'Oil spot' onycholysis, 67, 69
Old age, 6–7
  longitudinal lines, *49*, *50*
  onychogryphosis, 76
Omega nail, 183
'One hand–two foot' syndrome, 156
Onychatrophy, 42, *44–7*
Onychia punctata, 58
Onycho-dermal band, 3
Onychocryptosis, 172, 179–88
Onychodysplasia, index finger nails, 27, 39, 42
Onychodystrophy, 172
Onychogryphosis, 72, 174, 189, 201, 204–5
Onycholysis, 67–71, *67–9*, *71*, *143*, 144, *152*, 156, *156*, 178–9, *180*, 202–3
Onychomadesis, 56, *57*, 71–2, *73*, *74*, *170*, 178–9, *180*
Onychomatricoma, 81, 83
Onychomycosis, 10, 26, 69, 71, 76, 78, 83, 129, 135, 137, 146, 147, 155–68, *155–66*, 179, 201
Onychomycosis nigricans, 100
Onychophagia, 126
Onychophosis, 178, *179*
Onychoptosis defluvium, 72
Onychorrhexis, 50, 135
Onychoschizia, 63–5, *63*, *64*
Onychotillomania, 42, *47*, 87, 137, *187*, 205
Onychrogryphosis, 75, 76, *76*, 77
Opaque trachyonychia, 61
Orthopaedic devices, 178
Osler's disease, 23
Osteoarthritis, 27, 30, 110, 183, *191*

Osteoarthropathy, hypertrophic pulmonary, 19, 20
Osteochondroma, 99, 108
Osteoid osteoma, 21, 101, 194
Osteomalacia, 137
Osteomyelitis, 194
Osteoporosis, 137
Otopalatodigital syndrome, 34
Overcurvature, transverse, 26–30, *27–30*
Overlapping toes, *11*, 179

Pachydermoperiostosis, 19–20, *20*
Pachyonychia congenita, 27, 70, 78, 79, 93, 201
Painful nail, 193–5, *195–7*
Palmoplantar keratoderma, 83
Pancoast–Tobias syndrome, 23
Papilloma, subungual, 101, 194
Parakeratosis pustulosa, 60, 92, 93, 121, 128–30, *129*
Paraneoplastic acrokeratosis, 93
Parasitosis, 21
Paronychia:
  acute, 89–91, *90*, 126, 171, 194, *195*, *196*, 201–2
  chronic, 91–3, *93*, 125–6, *126*, 194, 202
  painful nail, 194
  pustulation, 121
  shedding, 72
  transverse lines, 56, 58
  trauma, 171, 187–8
  treatment, 201–2
Parrot beak nails, 35, *36*
Pellagra, 70, 146
Peloprenoic acid, 137
Pemphigoid, 124
Pemphigus, 72, 76, 92, 93
Pemphigus vulgaris, 61, 63
Penicillamine, 137, 151
Penicillin, 124, 125
Peptic ulcers, 83
Peripheral vascular disease, 87, 92
Periungal fibroma, 99
Periungual tissue disorders, 89–131, *90–130*
Periungual warts, 99–102, *99*, *101*, *102*, 205–6
Pernio, periostosis and lipo-dystrophy syndrome, 20
Perspiration, 15
Pertinax bodies, 4, 7

Peutz–Jeghers–Touraine syndrome, 101, 118, 147
Phenol, 186
Phenol red pH indicators, 163
Phenolphthalein, 151
Phenothiazines, 100, 151
Phospholipids, 200
Phosphorus poisoning, 23
Photo-onycholysis, 69, *69*, 70
Photochemotherapy, 70, 147, 203
Pigmentation, 3
  colour changes, 139
  malignant melanoma, 117–18
  onychomycosis, 157
  racial variations, 115, 118
Pilocarpine, 146
Pincer nails, 27–30, *27*, *28*, 78, 174, *182*, 183–5, *184*, *185*, 194
Pitting, 58–60, *58–61*, 128
Pityriasis rosea, 59, 60
Pityriasis rubra pilaris, 7, 75, 78, 83, 201
Pleonosteosis, 34
Plicatured nails, *27*, 30, *30*
Plummer–Vinson syndrome, 25
Pneumocystis carinii, 21
Pneumonia, 21
POEM syndrome, 23
Poisoning, 23, 146
Polycythaemia, 23
Polycythaemia vera, 65
Polydactyly, 37, 38–9
Porphyria, 26, 151
Porphyria cutanea tarda, 147
Potassium permanganate, 147, *151*
Prednisolone, 128
Prednisone, 202, 204
Preformed artificial nails, 200
Pregnancy, 70, 137, 147
'Press-on' nail polish, 200
Profile sign, clubbing, 19
Prosecutor's wart, 194
Prostheses, 201
Protein deficiency, 146
Proteoglycans, 200
Proteus, 100
Proteus syndrome, 38, *40*
Proximal nail fold, 1, 2, 3
  paronychia, 89, 91
Proximal subungual onychomycosis (PSO), 155, 157, *159*, 162, 167

Pruritic lymphoma, 42
Pruritus, 42
Pseudo-Hutchinson's sign, 117–18, 148, 190
Pseudo yellow nail syndrome, 27, *29*
Pseudoclubbing, 21, *22*, 34
Pseudocysts, myxoid, 50, *53*, 99, 101, 108–12, *110*, *111*, 191, *191*, 194
Pseudohypoparathyroidism, 34
Pseudoleukonychia, 146
Pseudomonas, 92, *152*, 200, 202, 203
Pseudomonas aeruginosa, 151, 202
Pseudomonas pyocyanea, 68
Pseudotumor, 21
Psoralens, 70, 116, 203
Psoriasis, 7, 129, 164–5
  arthropathy, 33
  Beau's lines, *56*, 57, *57*
  brachyonychia, *36*
  brittle nails, 136, 137
  hyperkeratosis, 72, *75*, *76*, 78
  koilonychia, 25, 26
  lamellar splitting, 65
  leukonychia, 144, 146
  longitudinal lines, 54
  nail abrasion, 201
  nail varnish, 200
  onychatrophy, 42, *45*
  onychogryphosis, 76
  onycholysis, 67, *68*, 69, 70, 71
  onychomadesis, *74*
  paronychia, 91, 92, 93, *95*
  and pincer nails, 30
  pitting, 59, *59*, 60, *61*, 128
  pustular, *45*, *74*, 126–7, *127*, *128*, 203, 204
  splinter haemorrhages, *81*, 83
  trachyonychia, 61
  treatment, 203–4
Psychotic episodes, 146
Pterygium, 42, 52, 83, 84–7, *85*, *86*, 171, *173*, 194
Pterygium inversum unguis, 85
Pulmonary disease, 83
Pulmonary fibrosis, 21
Punctate leukonychia, 141–2
Puretic syndrome, 34
Purple nails, 151
Purpura, subungual, 176

Pus, paronychia, 89–90, *90*, *196*
Pustular psoriasis, *45*, *74*, 126–7, *127*, *128*, 203, 204
Pustules, 121–31, *122*, *124–30*
PUVA, 70, 100, 126–7, 128, 203, 204
Pyogenic granuloma, 99, 100, 101, 105, 118, 171, *171*

Quarternary ammonium derivatives, 205
Quinine, 70
Quinine sulphate, 205

Racquet nail, *32*, 33, 34
Racquet thumb, 33
Radial artery puncture, 83
Radiation, longitudinal lines, 54
Radiodermatitis, 78, 87, 93, 115, 147, *196*
Radiotherapy, 85, 147, 203
Ragged cuticles, 93–6, *97*
Ram's horn deformity, 77
Raynaud's disease, 23, 26, 52, 83, 85, 86, 87, *145*, 194, 206
Recklinghausen's disease, 38
Recurring digital fibrous tumour of childhood (RDFT), 99, 105, 106, *106*
Red lines, 54
Red lunulae, *153*
Red nails, 151
Reiter's syndrome, 60, 70, 78, 91, 92, 93, 121, 128
Relapsing polychondritis, 7
Renal dialysis, 26, 84
Renal disease, 83, 146
Renal transplants, 146
Retinoic acid, 203
Retinoids, *64*, 65, 70, 72, 93, 126–7, 128, 203, 204
Rheumatic fever, 83
Rheumatoid arthritis, 49, 54, 83, 151
Ridges:
  herringbone, 53, *54*
  longitudinal, 52–3
  post–traumatic, 171, *172*
  transverse, *187*
Rippling, 58
Rosenau's depressions, 58
Rough nails, 59, 60–3, *61*, *62*

Rubinstein–Taybi syndrome, *31*, 33, 34

Sabouraud's medium, 163, *164*, 167
Salicylic acid, 203
'Salmon-patch' onycholysis, 67–9
Sarcoid dactylitis, 194
Sarcoidosis, 21, 23, 60, 83, 93, *96*
Sarcoma, 101
Scabies, Norwegian, 78
Scars, keloid, 102, 105
Schamroth, 19
Schuppli syndrome, 70
Scleroderma, *97*
Scopulariopsis brevicaulis, 80, 167
Sculptured artificial nails, 201
Scurvy, *82*, 83, 84
Scytalidium, 92, 167
Scytalidium dimidiatum, 116, 158, 167
Self-inflicted injury, *187*, 188, *188*, 189
Septicaemia, 83
Shedding, 71–2, *73*, *74*, 171, *188*, 189
Shiny nails, 13, 39–41, *41*
Shiny trachyonychia, 61–3
Shock, 146
Shoes, 10–15, *13*, *14*
  inserts, *12*, *192–3*
  microtrauma, 172–3, 174, *174*, 176–7, 178–9, *189*, 190
  pincer nails, 30
Short nails, *31–3*, 33–4, *35*
Sickle cell anaemia, 146
Silicon toe props, *12*
Silver, 100
Silver nitrate staining, *150*
Sneddon–Wilkinson disease, 127
Sodium hypochlorite, 202, 203
Sodium tetradecyl, 112
Soft nails, 133–7, 199–200
Soft tissue abnormalities, 67–87, *67–86*
Solehorn, 3
Spiegler tumours, 33, 34
Splinter haemorrhages, 80–3, *81*, *82*, 84, 170
Splinters, 171, 194

Splitting:
  brittle nails, 135, 136
  lamellar, 63–5, *63*, *64*, 135
  longitudinal, 52
  post-traumatic, 171, *172*
Spongiotic trachyonychia, 63
Spoon-shaped nails, 23–6, *24–6*
Sportsman's toe, 72, 176, *176*
Squamous cell carcinoma, 99, 100, 101, 113–14, 194
Squamous cells, 4
Squaric acid dibutylester (SADBE), 205
Staphylococci, 90
Staphylococcus aureus, 92, 171, 201, 202
Steroids, 202, 203, 204
Stevens–Johnson syndrome, 42, 56, 58, 72, 87, 93
Stick-on nail dressing, 200
Streptococci, 90, 124–5
Stub thumb, 34
Subtotal leukonychia, 141
Subungual exostosis, 99, 101, 108, *109*, 172, *174*
Subungual filamentous tumour, 101, 105–6
Subungual haematoma *see* Haematoma
Subungual hyperkeratosis, 72–80, *75–80*
Subungual melanotic lesions, 114–21, *114*, *115*, *117*, *119*
Subungual warts, 78, 99–102
Sulphaemoglobinaemia, 23
Sulphonamides, 146, 147
Sulphur, 4, 136
Sulphur deficiency syndromes, 133, 137
Sweat glands, 4
Sweating, 15
Swellings, 98–121
Sympathetic leukonychia, 146
Symphalangism, 38–9
Syphilis, 26, 58, 59, 60, 70, 72, 76, 92, 147
Syringomyelia, 23
Systemic sclerosis, 86, 87, 194

Tendon sheath, 191
Tendon sheath giant cell tumour, 99
Tennis toe, 176, 179
'Tented' nail, *174*
Terbinafine, 165
Terry's nail, 142, 144, 146

Tetracyclines, 70, 83, 147, 151
Thallium, 100, 146
Thiazide diuretics, 70
Thick nails, 72–80, *75–80*, 201
Thoracic tumours, 21
Thrombophlebitis, 76
Thumb:
  polydactyly, 38–9
  sucking, 92, 93, 121, 125–6, *126*, 129
Thymol, 203
Thyroid disease, 21, 26, 84, 147
Thyrotoxicosis, 70, 83
Tile-shaped nails, *27*, 30
Tinea cruris, *158*
Tinea pedis interdigitalis, 158, *160*
Toes:
  and foot function, 7–15
  foot shape, 10, *11*, *13*
  nail structure, 1, 3
  silicon props, *12*
Total leukonychia, 140–1, 146
Touraine, Solente and Golé syndrome, 20
Trachyonychia, 52, 59, 60–3, *61*, *62*
Transungual drug delivery system (TUDDS), 165
Transverse leukonychia, 141, *141*, *142*, 190, *190*
Transverse lines, 53–8, *55–7*
Transverse overcurvature, 26–30, *27–30*
Transverse ridges, *187*
Trauma:
  haematoma, 83, 119
  hyperkeratosis, 72, 78
  koilonychia, 26
  leukonychia, 146
  longitudinal grooves, 51, *51*, *52*, 54
  major trauma, 169–72, *169–74*
  melanonychia, 114, 115, 147
  microtrauma, 172–91, *175–91*
  nail shedding, 72
  onychogryphosis, 76
  onycholysis, 69, 70
  onychomadesis, *74*
  painful nail, 193–5, *195–7*
  paronychia, 89
  pitting, 59, 60
  pseudo-Hutchinson's sign, 118

pseudoclubbing, *22*
splinter haemorrhages, 82, 83
subungual exostosis, 108
transverse grooves, 57, 58
worn down nails, 42
Treatment, 199–206
Triamcinolone acetonide, 127, 203, 204
Trichinosis, 83
Trichophyton mentagrophytes var. interdigitale, 156, 158
Trichophyton rubrum, 77, 115–16, 156, *156*, 157, *158*, *159*, *164*
Trichophyton rubrum var. nigricans, 147, 157, 158
Trichophyton soudanense, 158, *161*, *164*
Trichothiodystrophy, 26
Tropical sprue, 21
Trumpet nail, *182*, 183
Trypaflavine, 70
Tuberculosis, 21
Tuberculosis cutis verrucosa, 99–100
Tuberous sclerosis, 38, 99, 103, *104*
Tumours, 98–121, *99–119*
  Bowen's disease, 112–13, *112*, *113*
  fibromas, 102–6, *103*, 194
  glomus tumour, 4, *53*, 54, 99, 101, 106–8, *107*, 151, 193, 194, *197*
  longitudinal lines, 50, *53*, 54
  malignant melanoma, 116–21, *117*, *119*

myxoid pseudocysts, 108–12, *110*, *111*
painful nail, 194
squamous cell carcinoma, 113–14
subungual exostosis, 108, *109*
thoracic, 21
warts, 99–102, *99*, *101*, *102*
Turf toe, 188
Turner's syndrome, 38
Twenty nail dystrophy, 59, 60, *62*, 63, 204

Ulcerative colitis, 23, 146
Unguis constringens, 27
Urea ointment, 204–5
Usure des ongles, *41*, 42
UV radiation, 6

Varicose veins, 76
Variola, 76
Vasculitis, 83, 84, 93, 194
Veillonella, 121, 123–4
Ventral pterygium, 84, 85, *86*, 87
Verruca vulgaris, 99, 105
Verrucous epidermal naevi, 101
Vesicles, 70
  herpes simplex, 122–3
  impetigo, 124
  Veillonella infection, 123–4
Vinyl chloride, 23
Viral warts, 99–102, *99*, *101*, *102*
Vitamin deficiencies, *82*, 137, 147

Vitamin E, 204
Vitiligo, 60
Volar digital nerves, 4, *5*

Walking, gait cycle, *8*, 9–10
Warfarin, 39, 151
Warts, 50, *57*, 70, 78, 99–102, *99*, *101*, *102*, 194, 205–6
Washboard nail plates, 51–2
'Watch-glass' deformity, 18, 19
Weed killers, 27
Wetting:
  brittle nails, 136
  hang nails, 96
  lamellar splitting, 65
  paronychia, 91, *93*
White nails, 140–6, *140–5*
White superficial onychomycosis (WSO), 155, 158, *160*, 162, *163*, 167
Whitlows, 23, 122, *122*, 125
Wilson's disease, 151
Worn down nails, 39–41, *41*, 189

X-rays, 72, 118, 171, 177, 195
Xanthoma, 101

Yellow nail syndrome, 7, 21, *22*, 27, *29*, 70, 72, 78, 93, 151, *152*, 204

Zidovudine, 116
Zinc deficiency, 56, 58, 93, *96*, 146